Here is the next best thing to spend̲
Professor Alan Thomas in his work ̲̲
informative and fascinating chapter provides an intro̲̲̲ ̲
seminar on psychiatric disorders and their treatments. Anchored
in medical expertise and a firm grasp of the holistic biblical
doctrine of the image of God, *Tackling Mental Illness Together*
exudes compassion and a deep conviction about the ministry
ordinary Christians can have to those who suffer.
Sinclair B. Ferguson, Professor of Systematic Theology, Redeemer
Theological Seminary, Dallas, Texas

Whether as professional, carer, family member or perhaps as a
patient, every one of us will have been affected by mental illness.
Christians may face further distress – is this behaviour sin or is it
sickness? From a biblical and medical framework, and using case
examples, consultant psychiatrist Alan Thomas makes everything
clear. Rational, readable and relevant, this book confirms that all
in Christian ministry and pastoral work can help tackle mental
illness.
Dr Andrew Fergusson, author, Hard Questions about Health and
Healing

Attitudes to mental illness today are still disfigured by too much
fear and too little understanding. Alan Thomas has written the
go-to resource for those who want to know more about this crucial
area. Firmly rooted in sound scholarship, it is nevertheless hugely
accessible to its target readership – pastors, clergy and all those
wanting to understand more about their own struggles or those
of a family member. Here, they will find the wisdom of reliable
clinical experience laced with academic rigour and good common
sense, all grounded in the word of God. I recommend it highly.
Glynn Harrison, speaker, author and a former professor of psychiatry

This easy-to-read book improves our understanding of common
mental health problems and their treatments. Using case studies
and biblical teaching, it also empowers us all to play our part in
helping by reminding us that little things (such as listening,
warmth and kindness) can help to improve the mental health
of those we encounter.
Debbie Hawker, clinical psychologist

Mental illness can have a devastating impact, and it is tempting for Christians to step back from efforts to help. Surely it's safer to 'leave it to the professionals'? Professor Alan Thomas, a consultant psychiatrist, disagrees. This is an accessible, practical, sensible and biblically grounded resource to help church leaders (and concerned church members) to navigate this challenging terrain.
Dr Sharon James, Social Policy Analyst, The Christian Institute

Professor Alan Thomas is a psychiatrist with research interests in brain imaging and molecular biology. But he believes that human beings are more than just physical matter. Rather, we are holistic combinations of material bodies and immaterial spirits / minds – what he calls 'psychosomatic wholes'. His book combines examples from his clinical practice, with summaries of scientific research and theological reflections on the Bible's teaching about the nature of humanity. The result is a comprehensive analysis of treatment possibilities for psychiatric disorders, presented in a way that will instil in church leaders the confidence to work together with mental health professionals to help people find healing from mental illness.
Nick Pollard, co-founder of EthosEducation.org and Chair of A Spiritual Path to Mental Health

This is a unique book, coming from a qualified, experienced and deeply thoughtful man, dealing with a subject demanding much insight, compassion and also plain speaking. Making a certain distinction between immoral behaviour and that which is the result of a disease of the mind can be at times perplexing. Every case seems to be uncharted territory. There have been occasions when we have needed help. To whom can we turn? Now my friend Alan Thomas has shared his own important insights with us in what will become a standard book on the subject, accessible and wise.
Geoff Thomas, author, editor, pastor and preacher, Alfred Place Baptist Church, Aberystwyth

ALAN THOMAS

TACKLING MENTAL ILLNESS TOGETHER

A biblical and practical approach

INTER-VARSITY PRESS
36 Causton Street, London SW1P 4ST, England
Email: ivp@ivpbooks.com
Website: www.ivpbooks.com

First published 2017

British Library Cataloguing-in-Publication Data
A catalogue record for this book is available from the British Library.

ISBN: 978-1-78359-559-4
eBook ISBN: 978-1-78359-560-0

Set in Dante 12/15 pt
Typeset in Great Britain by CRB Associates, Potterhanworth, Lincolnshire
Printed in Great Britain by Ashford Colour Press Ltd, Gosport, Hampshire

To Shona

CONTENTS

PREFACE

I've written and published a lot as a medical academic. But my previous publications were objective works of science. This book is personal. It is personal because people very close to me have suffered from mental illnesses, and it is hard not to let this colour what I've written. I hope that where this may have happened it will be for the better.

Another personal element is the range of examples of mental illness in this book. They are drawn from my experience – of people in churches and in the health service. But they are not transcripts. Details have been changed and cases merged to ensure that anonymity is preserved and no-one can be identified.

And it is personal because when writing every page I've been self-conscious that I'm airing my opinions. They are, others tell me, well-informed opinions. They are views I've discussed and been asked to write down for many years. Nonetheless, they are my views. They are not the kind of hard scientific statements I usually write. And at times I've been very conscious of simplifying and glossing over complex issues. Experts may be dissatisfied with some of what I've written. Read mercifully, dear friends, for simplifying to be clear for the intended general readership easily slips into over-simplification. My academic practice of nuanced argument and detailed proof has had to give way to streamlined clarity for what I hope is the greater good.

This takes me to the painful subject of references. My instinct and experience is to support every argument by biblical and scientific evidence. But this isn't that kind of book. Friends (see below) have encouraged me to remove many of the references to make it easier to read. And I have done so. I feel that what is left is a bit of a hotchpotch. Some statements are buttressed and others are not. I've tried to refer readers to other works and evidence where this will be helpful and/or the topic is controversial. You will judge how well I have succeeded.

And today I am very conscious of plagiarism. Recently (along with other academics) I've been warned about self-plagiarism. Here the criticism is making the same point in two different publications using the same words – even though they are my own words! I like to refer to other people's works where I am indebted to them. But to whom am I indebted? I really don't know how much of what I've written is 'original'. Probably nothing. I don't think any of the key arguments are. Many years ago I was debating with my father and made what I thought was a clever and original point. My dad nonchalantly replied that Bertrand Russell had said the same decades before. I've learned so much from so many people that it wouldn't be possible to acknowledge everyone (even if I could remember your contributions).

But there are some people who deserve acknowledgment for their specific contributions to this book. I would like to thank men in the Christian ministry who have read sections and contributed kind and constructive criticism to help shape this final version: Mark Richards, David Last, Gerard Hemmings and Stephen Rees. Two other friends in the ministry provided detailed and constructive criticism at several key stages in the gestation of this book: Mike Judge and Dan Peters. I'm grateful to all for helping me improve the focus of the book. I'm also indebted to the anonymous contributors to chapter 9. They have written movingly of their personal experiences of mental illness. The reader will understand why their contributions are anonymous. And I've benefited so much from the editorial experience of Eleanor Trotter at IVP who has greatly helped shape this for my target readership, and I am thankful to several anonymous reviewers for their comments which I'm sure have improved this final version.

Several friends nearer to home read over a chapter or two and provided valuable comments: Simon Calvert, Mike and Liz Davison, Mike Johnson, Rhys Curnow, Dr Grant Harris, James and Elspeth Grimwood and Dr Robert Smith. Dr Mandy Mackereth did a sterling job in reading many chapters and applying her medical and psychiatry experience to improving everything she touched. Dr Katherine Glover, a fellow consultant in old age psychiatry, read and critiqued several key chapters, and I'm grateful to her for helping keep my focus accurate and relevant. Finally, my debt to my beloved wife and fellow doctor Shona was already beyond description (certainly by this poor wordsmith). Throughout the long gestation and painful delivery of this book she has proven a magnificent midwife, providing the kind of candid advice and correction which only a wife can give. This final version, though, is one for which I bear responsibility, warts and all.

Most of all I am grateful to our God and Saviour Jesus Christ for blessing me with the necessary education, training and experience, and for granting me the health and strength to complete this book: 'You may say to yourself, "My power and the strength of my hands have produced this wealth for me." But remember the LORD your God, for it is he who gives you the ability' (Deuteronomy 8:17–18). My prayer throughout has been that he would make it useful to church leaders so they might be better equipped to help those needy people with mental illnesses in our midst. To him be the glory for ever, Amen.

INTRODUCTION:
SETTING THE SCENE

'You should write a book, Alan,' he said, 'to help ministers like me.' That was too long ago, after an extended conversation about how he could understand and help a suffering believer with a mental illness in his church. It nagged away at me. But here finally is the fruit of that suggestion. This book aims to help not just Christian ministers but all those in formal and informal leadership in churches.

It is written with the conviction that such people are well equipped to provide help to those with mental illnesses. Recently in the field of psychiatry there has been a trend towards recognizing that people with minimal training can provide real therapeutic benefit to the mentally ill. I'm convinced that mature Christian men and women have the necessary skills and experience to provide such benefit to the many people with mental illnesses in our churches.

Mental illnesses are devastating

For mental illnesses are common. We all have people in our churches with them. And they are devastating because they strike at those qualities which make us human. Consequently, across societies and throughout history they have been recognized as a terrible affliction. They have borne a variety of labels: broader ones like 'madness' and 'insanity', and narrower terms such as 'melancholia' and 'dementia'. Andrew Scull, a historian of psychiatry and Professor at the University of California, comments,

> Madness – massive and lasting disturbances of behaviour, emotion, and intellect . . . lunacy, insanity, psychosis, mental illness – whatever term we prefer, its referents are disturbances of reason, the passions, and human action that frighten, create chaos . . . that mark a gulf between the common-sense reality most of us embrace, and the discordant version some humans appear to experience.[1]

Pulpit and pew

And mental illnesses do not discriminate. They afflict people of all races, all social classes, male and female, rich and poor. They afflict church ministers and church members. No-one is exempt. I've included examples throughout the book to aid interest and understanding. These are drawn from real people. They are, of course, carefully anonymized, as I said in my Preface. You may think you see someone you know. That is fine. But it won't be the person I was thinking about! Mental illnesses are common and patterns recur, and so similarities will frequently happen by chance. So if you make such a link, it will be the wrong person. But it will probably help your understanding. Most of the examples in this book are from 'the pew', but men in the pulpit have also written of their own struggles with mental illness.

Timothy Rogers, a Puritan minister, was unable to serve as a pastor for eight years at the end of the seventeenth century because he was incapacitated by a severe depressive illness. In those days this was termed 'melancholy', and he wrote movingly of his depression and his inability to rid himself of it:

> It is commonly said by others who do not know what melancholy is, 'Why do you think . . . so much? Divert yourselves; think of something else.' But it is no more possible for people, where this disease comes with violence, to divert their thoughts than it is possible for a man . . . who has a broken arm or leg [to] walk and act as he used to do before . . .
>
> . . . it is as natural for a melancholy person to fear, and to meditate on terror, as it is for a sick man to groan, or for one in health to breathe. It is certain that . . . melancholy will not be relieved by mere words or sentences; they cannot indeed cast out their troubled thoughts; they cannot turn away their minds; they can think of nothing but what they do think just as a man with a toothache cannot forbear to think of his pain . . . Though others urge us to rule our thoughts, it gives no relief, but only adds to our misery to be frequently urged to do that which we cannot do.[2]

Nothing new

So mental illnesses are not, as is sometimes implied, a recent invention. And the care of the mentally ill has often been appalling. For example, in 1817 an Irish MP investigating the care of the mentally ill lamented,

> There is nothing so shocking as madness in the cabin of the Irish peasant . . . When a strong man or woman gets the

complaint, the only way they have to manage is by making
a hole in the floor of the cabin, not high enough for the person
to stand up in, with a crib over it to prevent his getting up. This
hole is about five feet deep, and they give this wretched being
his food there, and there he generally dies.[3]

And during this same period in Germany a physician wrote,

It is a remarkable sensation to come from the bustle of a big
city into one of these madhouses . . . fools who laugh without
reason and fools who torture themselves without reason. Like
criminals we lock these unfortunate creatures into mad-cages,
into antiquated prisons, or put them next to the nesting holes
of owls in desolate attics over the town gates, or in the damp
cellars of the jails, where the sympathetic gaze of a friend of
mankind might never behold them; and we leave them there,
gripped by chains, corrupting in their own filth.[4]

These anecdotes are a salutary reminder of the grim reality
of untreated mental illness. The history of mental illness is
the history of such poor, afflicted people. They were cast out
of society, becoming tramps and vagrants, mocked as village
idiots and locked up in back rooms, chained to posts in barns
or despatched by families to madhouses and asylums. Before
the advent of modern medicines and the rise of asylums,
mental illness was indeed encountered in all its raw horror.

Mental illnesses remain devastating. Depressive illness is
the third largest cause of disability in the world and the largest
in wealthy countries. People with schizophrenia and bipolar
disorder die about fifteen years younger than everyone else.
This is largely due to poor physical health and not to suicide.
Anxiety and eating disorders also increase death rates (by
40%–90%), so sufferers die at a younger age.

At a national level mental illness is very expensive. The King's Fund estimates that by 2026 the cost to England alone for anxiety illnesses will be over £14 million every year and over £12 million for depression. Dementia will cost England £35 million every year. If dementia were a company, it would be the largest in the world, having more revenue than even Walmart or Apple. But the personal devastation of mental illnesses is not captured with such figures.

UK evangelist Roger Carswell wrote in *Where Is God in a Messed-up World?* of his perplexity when he was struck down by depression. He knew he was changing, struggling to cope with the work he once enjoyed, and searching to understand what was going on. Had he done something wrong? Was he being afflicted for some sin or sins? He couldn't identify any, and continued to worsen:

> I began to find certain aspects of my work overwhelming. Every phone call seemed too much for me and I couldn't cope with inconsequential chatter, or even the laughter of others. I became annoyed even when people asked me to preach somewhere (which is my beloved life's work!) . . . I was beginning to sink into a depth of great, inward darkness. I did not want to talk with anyone. I continued to regularly have my devotions and go to church, but avoided meeting with people at the end of the service . . . My mind was telling me things that were not true . . . I believed nobody cared whether I lived or died. I went to bed each evening hoping I would die in the night, and would wake up the next day feeling I could not face the hours ahead. However, even in my lowest moments I was convinced that God was in control of all that was going on . . . Although I don't generally drink alcohol, in the darkness of my depression I wanted to get drunk. I thought that if I was drunk, at least for an evening I would not feel the tangible,

emotional pain that was within . . . As a Christian, I am sure
it is not wrong to be on medication. The fall has wrecked our
beings, and we can be affected physically and mentally. As I
would not hesitate to take medication if I was physically sick,
so I was relaxed to take medication for my mind.[5]

Eventually, after trying a few antidepressants, he saw a psychiatrist who found the right medication to get him well again.
But he knows that depression frequently recurs and comments,
'Frankly, I would fear it happening and would not wish the
inward darkness on anyone, but I am also aware that God
works all things together for my good and his glory.'[6]

Reading this book

This book is best read from beginning to end, of course. It is
arranged in order to build an understanding of mental illness
so we then know how to help those with such illnesses. In
chapter 1 we begin by thinking about who we are as human
beings. We have minds. Is mental illness something that just
affects our minds? Or does it involve our bodies too? Think of
Jesus in Gethsemane. As he contemplated Calvary and his
suffering there, the mental stress powerfully affected his body.
It was a cold spring night; fires were needed to keep warm.
But such was the impact on his body of his mental anguish
that he sweated profusely (Luke 22:39–46).[7] Our minds affect
our bodies. And vice versa.

In chapter 2 we reflect on the implications of being created
in God's image. Roger Carswell vividly describes the total
impact of his illness, doesn't he? His thinking, decision-
making and perception of himself and the world around him
were distorted by his depression. Depression is not just about
feelings. So what is it? And what is mental illness anyway? We

tackle these vital questions in chapter 3 where we learn how mental illness differs from distress and from bad behaviour.

Having understood what we mean by mental illness (and what we don't!), we want to know how to help. And to help we need to know why. We are not to be like Tennyson's 600 in the Light Brigade charging into battle. Ours is to reason why. Why is he sick? Is it her fault? Why did this happen to me? The mind is complex and much of its activity is unconscious. So in chapter 4 we look at what the Bible teaches about the unconscious mind and learn of its relevance to mental illness. And we look at what Freud said too.

In chapter 5 we consider how various types of stress impact on our minds and bodies to cause mental illnesses. We learn important lessons from the history of shell shock and hysteria. We also touch briefly on the hugely important influence of the brain (and thus neurobiological mechanisms). This chapter concludes with a model for understanding mental illness that shows how we can help.

Chapters 6 and 7 deal with the treatment and care of people with mental illness. One day after I became a consultant psychiatrist I was unexpectedly told that one of 'my' patients had raped someone. Even today my colleagues are amused when they learn that my consultant career began with such a problem. And I use inverted commas because of course I hadn't yet met him. My first encounter was when he was under arrest. I was asked if he was guilty. Or did his mental illness 'let him off'? In chapter 6 we grasp this thorny issue of personal responsibility.

Chapter 7 reviews the main kinds of treatments used in psychiatry. Sadly, each has been challenged as ineffective and/or immoral. Including by Christians. So we learn how the Bible's teaching on wine justifies our use of medication and how church leaders can use talking treatments to help too. We conclude with a framework for helping people with mental illness, discussing the important role for church leaders and churches themselves.

We all know the importance of practising what we preach. We all watch and learn from one another's behaviour. It is a very effective way of learning. And so in chapters 8 and 9 we conclude by learning from actual examples. Rather than describing different mental illnesses, I have chosen to illustrate them. And then I give some explanations of the ways psychiatric services seek to help such people and how we in churches can help too.

Begin at the beginning . . . or the end

So how should you read this book? You may be tempted to jump to the final two chapters full of examples of mental illnesses and so begin at the end. If you do so, fair enough. But please do then go back and read the rest. The earlier chapters introduce important ideas and lay out a framework for understanding mental illnesses, culminating in the stress-vulnerability model at the end of chapter 5. They also provide insights through other examples of how we can help the mentally ill.

The take-home message

At medical school I knew a student who would doze, or perhaps even sleep, through each lecture. But when the lecturer uttered the magic words, 'Now, the take-home message is . . .', he would open his eyes, pick up his pen and write down these key summary points. So, in memory of that man and as one who knows him as well as himself, each chapter of this book concludes with a bullet-point summary of the key issues. So for this chapter . . .

Key chapter points

- Mental Illnesses are devastating because they damage us body and soul, impairing key aspects of our image-ness (chapters 1 and 2).
- Mental illnesses are very common, but defining mental illness is important for distinguishing mental illnesses from life's distresses, and from bad behaviour (chapter 3).
- Unconscious and conscious factors contribute to mental illnesses and help us to understand and help those who suffer from them (chapters 4 and 5).
- We help the mentally ill by working with them as responsible image-bearers and by working with the treatments used by specialist health services (chapters 6 and 7).
- The different types of mental illness may be usefully grouped into two main categories, which form the content of chapters 8 and 9.

1. IT'S NOT ALL IN THE MIND

The court was amazed. The judge had acquitted her of adultery. But how could he have done when she was pregnant and her husband had been away for four years? He ruled that she had become pregnant through her mind when she had dreamed about her husband during his absence! This was in Grenoble in 1637,[1] and the fact that such a decision could be made at all illustrates the widespread acceptance that the mind could produce substantial changes in the body.

No such ruling would be made today. Neuroscience and psychiatry are heavily influenced by materialism, with its assumption that humans have no mind distinguishable from the body. The mind/soul was once acknowledged as a real and powerful entity. Now it is conceived as a mere by-product of the brain. The brain, it has been said, secretes the soul as the gall bladder secretes bile.

The Bible teaches that the mind/soul is a real entity distinguishable from the physical body and not merely a product of the workings of the brain. But also, these two components, the body and the mind/soul, are normally joined together, interacting in the whole human person. As we attempt to construct a biblical approach to mental illness, it is important we consider human nature. Mental illness is not all in the mind. Nor is it all in the brain. It involves both. Together.

The myth of organic mental illness

Thomas Szasz was an anti-psychiatry psychiatrist. He initiated a fallacy that has often been repeated in Christian circles, especially in the writings of Jay Adams and those who followed him. Szasz claimed, against all historical and scientific evidence, that mental illness was a fiction, a construct created by society to label and dispose of people who are inconvenient. He asserted that all illness was physical and recognized only organic brain disease.

Following this Szaszian line, Adams stated,

> Organic malfunctions affecting the brain that are caused by brain damage, tumors, gene inheritance, glandular or chemical disorders, validly may be termed mental illnesses. But at the same time a vast number of other human problems have been classified as mental illnesses for which there is no evidence they have been engendered by disease or illness at all.[2]

And elsewhere he asserted, 'Psychiatry's legitimate function is to serve those who suffer from organic difficulties.'[3]

Adams followed Szasz and the anti-psychiatrists in propagating the idea that there was a distinction between genuine 'organic illness' and 'mental illness'. The latter was behaviour conveniently labelled as 'mental illness' in order to excuse people from sin. Genuine mental illness had to be physical, due to brain disease. Any other kind of aberrant behaviour, lacking such a clear physical basis, is not illness at all but moral deviance (for some Christians) or societal labelling (for the anti-psychiatrists).[4] There is no place, then, for mental illness due to stressful life events or suffering at the hands of others.

Alzheimer's and Parkinson's diseases – not real illnesses?

Sticking rigidly to this 'organic brain disease' approach would mean that both Alzheimer's disease and Parkinson's disease would historically have been denied the status of 'real' illnesses. People exhibiting 'the shaking palsy' (now known as Parkinson's disease), who saw their doctor because of trembling and a funny walk, would have been dismissed as merely 'behaving strangely'. They did not have a real illness because no organic cause was then known. When they became depressed or started hallucinating (both common in Parkinson's disease), this would simply have confirmed the behavioural and moral nature of their problem. However, once the brain pathology was identified by Frederic Lewy in 1912, then, miraculously, what had been 'behavioural' became a 'real disease'! Now sufferers had a real illness and could be spared the opprobrium of having merely a behavioural or moral problem.

In 1905 Auguste D was the first person to be formally diagnosed as having Alzheimer's disease. But when she saw her psychiatrist, her main symptoms were mental. She had hallucinations and depression and memory problems. She would have been dismissed by those of a Szaszian/Adams persuasion as merely a troubled person whom society wished to label as sick. Fortunately for her, Alzheimer and his colleagues rightly diagnosed her as having a dementia. They recognized her hallucinations and depression as part of this dementia. And when she died, Alois Alzheimer examined her brain tissue under his microscope and identified the brain disease which now bears his name. Again, the advances of science converted 'behavioural problems' into real illnesses, due to real diseases.

Of course, Thomas Szasz, Jay Adams and others have always been willing to acknowledge that Alzheimer's disease and Parkinson's disease are 'genuine illnesses', due to 'real diseases'. But this is only because the evidence of brain disease was already established when they propounded their views. Clinically, though, such diseases would have been indistinguishable from other forms of 'madness' in the nineteenth and early twentieth centuries. And as science has advanced further during the twentieth and into the twenty-first centuries, other 'non-diseases' have been elevated to 'genuine illness' status.

People suffering from other historical forms of 'madness', like schizophrenia, melancholia (severe depression) and manic depression (bipolar disorder), have now been shown to have a major genetic contribution. Many neuroimaging studies have reported clear abnormalities in the structure of the brain tissue and aberrant patterns in brain function. Along with other academic researchers, I have also demonstrated tissue changes under the microscope (in the size and number of brain cells) in people with these mental illnesses. It is now widely accepted that these and other mental illnesses, like Parkinson's disease and Alzheimer's disease, have brain pathology and are therefore 'real' diseases. For families, psychiatrists and others who have cared for such people this is not surprising. The severity and pattern of the disturbances they have endured have always shown they were sick. Adams's approach conflicts with a wealth of evidence about the basis and causation of mental illness. But more importantly, his approach to mental illness contradicts the Bible.

Mind and brain (body and soul or vice versa)

God created Adam using material from his physical creation (dust of the earth) and he then breathed life into this substance to make Adam a living being (Genesis 2:7). Animals are also called 'living creatures'.[5] What marks Adam out, though, is the close personal involvement of God in fashioning him from the dust. He artistically shapes him and mouth-to-mouth breathes life into his physical body.

This passage emphasizes our wholeness. These verses do not explicitly teach that humans have two components, body and soul. But the fact that Adam is made from both the dust of the earth and the 'breath of life' suggests these two elements. What the 'breath of life' specifically refers to may not be clear in the Genesis account, but it is clear from the rest of Scripture. We have two parts, a material element (body) and an immaterial element (spirit, often called 'soul', and used interchangeably with mind).

In the Bible we are taught that the soul/spirit is able to exist without the body and fully capable of engaging in the worship of God. The glorified spirits in heaven are not shown as floating, lifeless entities. Rather, we read of the souls of Christians in heaven calling out to the Lord (Revelation 6:9–10), which shows they retain their mental faculties. Jesus reassured the dying and now believing thief that that very day they would be together in paradise (Luke 23:43). This shows he understood his human spirit/soul would be taken to heaven at the time of his bodily death where the thief would join him. The disembodied thief would continue to enjoy his personal relationship with the Lord Jesus Christ. Similarly, Stephen, at the time of his death, committed himself to his Saviour, saying, 'Lord Jesus, receive my spirit' (Acts 7:59).

From these texts we infer that all the faculties needed for worship are retained in the disembodied soul. Although the spirit/soul can function without the body and perform all these uniquely human abilities, the opposite, it appears, is not true. The body without the spirit is dead (James 2:26). When the soul/spirit departs from the body at death, the tent left behind is lifeless and has no residual faculties with which to worship. The corpse has no capacity to serve God.

A psychosomatic whole

My children ridicule me: 'You're not going on about psycho-somatic wholes again, are you, Dad?' 'Yes,' I reply, 'because it is important.' The phrase brings together two biblical (Greek) words for mind/soul (*psyche*) and body (*soma*). And the term 'psychosomatic' is used in medicine. Thus, I feel doubly justified in using this phrase! It captures the vital truth that we are created from material and non-material elements, a body and a soul joined together. This is our proper condition. Theologian Michael Horton comments, 'Whilst the body and soul *can* be separated, they are not *meant* to be separated, and our salvation is not complete until we are bodily raised as whole persons (Romans 8:23).'[6] Paul does not want to be naked. He wants to be clothed with his 'heavenly dwelling', his resurrection body (2 Corinthians 5:4). The naked state of souls in heaven is suboptimal, a temporary consequence of the fall while we await the end of the age and the resurrection of the dead.

Wholly ill

So the Bible's teaching is clear. We are psychosomatic wholes. When we are ill, we are ill in our bodies and in our minds. You don't get one without the other. Obviously mental illnesses involve the mind. But they also affect the body. Margaret has a chronic version of schizophrenia. You can see this in her flat, expressionless face and her awkward movements. David has dementia that is wasting his body and leaving him more stooped and stiff every day. William has depression and his body now hardly moves at all, and he too is wasting away.

But what about physical illnesses? These are bodily illnesses, but guess what, they also affect the mind. When you have flu it doesn't just affect your body, does it? A materialistic flu virus doesn't say to itself, 'I can only make the body ill here because there is no mind.' When ill you can't concentrate to think properly. You are emotional and struggle to make decisions because your mind is ill too.

You may not have heard of myxoedema madness. Googling will give you 5,580 hits (today anyway). It was caused by a severe disease of the thyroid gland in the neck. Today this illness (now called hypothyroidism) is almost always identified by blood tests for thyroid hormones at a very early stage. It is effectively treated by the prescription of thyroxine tablets which replace the deficient hormones. Historically, however, myxoedema caused a wide range of symptoms. Some were physical, such as greasy hair, weight gain, cold skin and goitre (enlarged thyroid gland). But others were mental. It caused sadness, poor concentration, deranged thinking and eventually dementia. It also caused hallucinations and delusions – key symptoms of psychosis and the hallmarks of 'myxoedema madness'. All illness is psychosomatic.

What are we made of?

But what is soul? What are we made from? The Bible doesn't address such questions. It teaches us about human behaviour and relationships. Michael Horton observes, 'Just as biblical faith does not speculate on the "whatness" of God's hidden essence but on the "whoness" (i.e., the character, actions and purposes) revealed in the script, the same may be said of the way in which that faith describes humanity.'[7] The Scriptures deal with how we are to live and relate to God and other people ('whoness' issues). They do not tell us what substance we are made from. But doesn't the Bible have lots of words about the different parts of human beings? Yes. But we need to handle them with care.

In the Old Testament no fewer than eighty different words are used for parts of us related to our emotion and behaviour.[8] The four commonest are: 'heart', 'liver', 'kidney' and 'bowels'. But their meanings all overlap. 'Heart' has the widest range of meaning. It frequently refers to the core of our being, combining our will, our intellect and our emotions. But I don't have a special part of my soul which is 'heart'. Nor are there other parts of my mind / soul which are 'kidneys' or 'bowels'. These words were clearly derived from physical anatomy. Perhaps it was thought that the properties of thinking, feeling and willing were located in these bodily organs. But I doubt it. Anyway, these words should not be read this way.

These words in the Bible do not describe distinct elements. Human beings are not built as it were of bricks labelled 'heart', 'kidneys' and so on:

> These several words do not . . . characterise man as a
> compound of separate and distinct elements. Hebrew
> psychology does not divide up man's nature into mutually
> exclusive parts. Behind these usages of words the thought
> conveyed by the Genesis account that man's nature is twofold
> remains.[9]

We know human beings are twofold (body and soul/spirit) because of the explicit biblical teaching summarized above, not because of the semantics of the biblical words.

It would be a great mistake to attempt to construct from such words 'an anatomy of the soul'. And a great mistake to try to work out whether a mental illness was due to damage to some such alleged part of the mind/soul. As if 'sadness of heart', for example, teaches us that depression is due to damage to the heart part of the soul. Ironically, there is a lot of research evidence (including some of mine) that depression is related to (physical) heart disease! This fits with us being psychosomatic wholes. All illness is holistic.

How do body and soul work together?

We are not given any explicit biblical teaching on how the body and soul/spirit work together. There are good reasons, however, for regarding the body and soul as acting in union so that what happens in the body has something corresponding happening in the spirit/soul.

The Scriptures show that our souls/spirits know and learn (Isaiah 29:24; Mark 2:8; 1 Corinthians 2:11), express feelings of distress (John 13:21; Acts 17:16), sadness (Proverbs 17:22) and joy (Psalm 35:9; Isaiah 61:10), and have desires or drives to do things, to will or make decisions (1 Samuel 1:15; Psalm 84:2). Science has shown there are linked brain areas that form circuits for different thinking processes. And other circuits for feelings (emotions). And others for perceptual and volitional processes.

It seems reasonable in the light of the biblical emphasis on our wholeness that these brain circuits correspond to these rational, emotional, perceptual and volitional processes in the soul referred to in these Scriptures. It would be peculiar if, for example, when our brain circuitry operates to recall information, process it and reason from it, there were no corresponding thinking processes in the soul. Our behaviour is holistic, involving the smooth and harmonious union of body and soul/spirit. Our behaviour involves our thoughts (the cognitive or intellectual element of our behaviour), our feelings (the emotional element), our perception (awareness of outside ourselves) and our will (the volitional element). And it is the whole person who thinks, feels, perceives and acts.

When someone is mentally ill, we may identify abnormalities in their brain circuitry and aim to correct these. But we can deduce that there are parallel and linked changes in the soul, derangements of perception and feeling and so on. We don't know how this linkage works, but the reality of this linkage should inform our approach to mental illness.

When Colin became depressed, he entered our research study. His brain imaging revealed the expected (subtle) abnormalities in brain areas associated with depression. And his blood tests showed chemical (steroid hormone) changes in his body and evidence of heart disease. These changes were linked to his brain abnormalities and his depression. Of course, we had no scan or chemical tests for his soul. But we did do tests of his intellect and emotions. These showed abnormalities that were consistent with the brain changes on his scan and steroid changes in his body. He was affected by his depression in different interrelated parts of his body and his soul. Colin was ill with his depression as a whole being, as a psychosomatic whole.

Job and his illness

Did Job in the Old Testament have a depressive illness? Many have claimed that he did. The danger here, however, is coming to the Bible to make it answer questions God never intended us to ask. There have been many interpretations of Job. But I don't think that anyone has claimed it should be read as a psychiatry textbook! What do we actually read? Job was afflicted with 'loathsome sores from the sole of his foot to the crown of his head' (Job 2:7 ESV). So he had a skin disease, not a mental illness!

However, as a consequence of this physical illness and, importantly, also from the stress from his multiple bereavements and social ostracism, Job developed depressive symptoms. His mood became low, his thinking became negative, he lost weight and his sleep was disturbed. It isn't clear he had a depressive illness. But he did have mental symptoms characteristic of depression. Job was ill with physical and mental symptoms. And these resulted from a combination of physical (skin disease) and psychological elements (bereavement, alienation from society).

From the biblical data we would expect that any 'organic illness' would have mental symptoms, and any 'mental illness' would have organic or physical features. And, as doctors know, this is precisely what we do find. Oxford Professor of Psychiatry Tom Burns states,

> Psychiatrists . . . point to the frequency of physical symptoms in mental illnesses (pain and tiredness) and mental symptoms in physical illnesses (depression, anxiety, hallucinations) . . . One of the reasons for the under-diagnosis of psychiatric problems in general practice is that psychological symptoms are part and parcel of most physical illness.[10]

Within medicine there is a group of disorders which are usually referred to as 'psychosomatic illnesses' because in these the interaction of body and soul is especially obvious.

By convention some lie within psychiatry, for example anxiety disorders, and some within general medicine, for example fibromyalgia and irritable bowel syndrome. But an adequate approach to understanding and treating such illnesses requires a holistic approach, which we will discuss in chapters 7–9.

In fact, it is impossible to think of a physical illness that does not affect the mind. And the opposite is also true. There is no mental illness that does not affect the body. Core features of depression include fatigue, weight loss and problems with bodily movement ('psychomotor retardation', a phrase that points to this influence of mind on body). Similarly, schizophrenia is associated with changes in bodily posture and movement.[11] Anxiety disorders cause difficulties with breathing, tingling of the skin, abdominal discomfort, changes in the heartbeat and so on. And, more expectedly perhaps, we've seen how true this is also for dementia. Thus, whichever way we look at illnesses, whether as primarily physical or primarily mental, we see that they will always impact the whole person. We saw this in the cases of Margaret, David, William and Colin.

The impact of the curse

Adam was created as a psychosomatic whole. But when he sinned, he and the whole creation were cursed. The consequences of the fall were not restricted to human beings. Or even to the physical creation. All creation, visible and invisible, was cursed (Romans 8:19–23; Ephesians 1:20–21). So both body and soul are now corrupted by the effects of God's judgment on Adam's sin. Here I don't mean corrupted morally, but materially: the 'substance' of the soul, like that of the body, was damaged by sin and the consequent curse by God.

We are familiar with ageing and sickness in the body. We know that this is a result of the curse. But Adam fell as a whole being, body and soul. And he was cursed as a whole. His body and soul together were corrupted and damaged. And in him we all were subjected to weakness and corruption (Romans 5:12) along with the rest of creation (Romans 8:20–22). Our spirit/soul was not exempted. Those properties we tend to attribute to the soul were corrupted. We've seen that these properties also reside in the brain. But whether regarded from the material side of the brain, or the immaterial side of the spirit/soul, they are now weakened and corrupted. Our corrupted, decaying body is accompanied by a corrupted and decaying soul. Hence mental illness has become part of cursed creation.

Harry is frequently off sick. But he isn't lazy. And I would say he is mentally strong. It is just that every time a bug goes around, he gets it and he gets it badly. We don't fully understand this. As a result of factors such as a better immune system and a more robust physical constitution, some of us catch the same bug and carry on fairly normally while others like Harry are laid low in bed.

Other people are weaker mentally. Their mental faculties are more damaged and so they are less resilient to stress. We all know that James is readily destabilized mentally (rationally, emotionally and so on). He became emotionally labile and weepy and unable to reason clearly when his son failed an exam and when his wife didn't get promoted. We know he has a fragile soul/mind. And he needs extra understanding and care. But this is just the soul/mind equivalent of Harry's bodily weakness, isn't it?

This variability in people's mental strength has long been recognized through the use of now 'incorrect' terms like 'neurotic' and 'weak nerves' for those more vulnerable to distress and mental illness. We seem to find it easier to accept that some people are weaker bodily than to accept that some are weaker in their spirits/souls. But both are consequences of the fall and curse, with some of us having more physical damage and some having more soul damage.

In arguing like this I realize the danger of encouraging us to think of human beings as composed of separate parts, body and soul. But I hope I've made clear by now the importance of our fundamental psychosomatic wholeness. However, I also want to encourage an approach to mental illness that does not consciously or unconsciously restrict to the body the damage arising from the curse. We need to recognize that illness arises from both mental/psychological and physical causes. For further biblical understanding of mental illness and its holistic nature, we will require a complementary perspective on who we are as human beings and why we become ill. We need to consider the Bible's teaching on our creation in God's image.

Key chapter points

- Humans are psychosomatic wholes (body and soul united).
- Soul/mind and body are continuously and intimately interacting.
- All illnesses involve the body and the mind/soul.
- No mental illnesses affect only the mind.

2. RULE AND RELATIONSHIP

He was chatting away with his back to me when I first approached him. But no-one else was there. He was talking to the wall in front of him. Or so it appeared. Really he was talking to his hallucinations, to the voices he engaged with most of the time. And he was a mess. Literally, because he was dishevelled, smelly and dirty. His speech when we talked was incoherent.

We brought him into hospital to restart his drugs: antipsychotics for his schizophrenia. But he didn't stay long. The nurses let him walk out the door; no-one wanted him to stay. I think some regarded him as not truly human. Certainly he was not treated with kindness and respect.

Are such individuals with mental illness fully human? Do they bear the image of God like the rest of us? The Nazi party in 1930s Germany said 'no'. And so such inmates of German asylums were among the first to be eliminated by the National Socialist Party 'Archive of Race Hygiene'. 'Mercy deaths', by starvation, shooting and other means, were combined with compulsory sterilization.[1] The programme for the systematic elimination of the mentally ill was promptly implemented by the Medical Inspectorate of the Waffen SS wherever the German army conquered.[2]

Unfortunately, this is not merely a grim historical truth. In the UK and other countries people with dementia and mental handicap now find themselves in the cross-hairs of the 'death with dignity' (aka euthanasia) movement. Given half a chance, the man at the start of the chapter and those like him would be killed (mercifully, of course).

After all, such people have 'lost their minds'. And is reason not necessary to be fully human? Or, in scriptural terms, the image of God resides in our mental faculty, doesn't it? The Nazis weren't right then, were they? What exactly does the Bible mean by the image of God, and how does this relate to mental illness?

Whole persons in God's image

In Genesis 1:26–27 we are told that God created us in his own image and likeness. This 'image-ness' or likeness is true of us as whole creatures. The two Hebrew words for image and likeness overlap in meaning and both refer to the whole human being.[3]

We are not told that only some part of us is made in God's image. No. Each as a whole *is* God's image-bearer. Gordon Wenham observes, 'The OT does not sharply distinguish the spiritual and material . . . The image of God must character-ise man's whole being, not simply his mind or soul on the one hand or his body on the other.'[4] Similarly, theologian Herman Bavinck stated, 'Man does not just bear or have the image of God but is the image of God and that . . . image of God extends to man in his entirety.'[5]

Our abilities to think and communicate, and even to self-reflect, are not quite uniquely human. They exist in a perfected and greater form in God. But they do distinguish us from all other creatures in this world. Our capacity to experience emotion, and to sense the feelings of others as we relate to them, mirrors qualities in God. Our power to determine a course of action and to fulfil that purpose replicates in a tiny way the power and actions of the Almighty himself. And such qualities are holistic. Thinking or feeling is not located in some special part of us. We think or feel as whole human beings.

Holistic implications

It is important to recognize the holism of our divine image. This image is not found in a single quality (or a few qualities) of human beings. It is not located in some part of us that may be lost. Rather, we maintain that each human actually is God's image. Even the most severely mentally ill retain the image of God. My patient with schizophrenia, so distorted in his thinking and damaged in his perception of the world, has not lost God's image. A woman with severe dementia has not crossed some line where she has lost God's image. This is not possible. To be human is to be God's image. Mental illness damages our thinking, our emotions, our volition and our relationships. But it can never erase our image-ness.

Relationships are us

The Bible tells us that, as God's image-bearers, we were given two major functions by God: to rule the earth (Genesis 1:26–28) and to relate to other humans (Genesis 2:18–24). Rule and relationship are how we express his image. Of course, our primary relationship is with God himself. We are to be heavenward in our orientation as we carry out these functions in his service.

God himself is eternally personal, indeed tri-personal. He exists in three persons, the Father, the Son and the Holy Spirit, known as the Trinity, who live in loving relationships within the Godhead. So, as God's image-bearers, we are personal. All men and women bear God's image and therefore reflect his personal and interpersonal qualities in modified, finite form.

Adam walked with God in the Garden of Eden, a close personal relationship. Earlier, in Genesis 1:26 we read the intriguing words: 'Let us . . . in our image'. These plural pronouns teach us immediately that our divine image is derived from a plurality of persons. God speaks of the Godhead using the first person plural ('us' and 'our'). A fellowship. Not an individual. It may be too much to infer the doctrine of the Trinity from Genesis 1:26, but in the light of later biblical revelation, it is best understood as the Father, Son and Spirit conferring and working together. And so we are prepared for 'that they may rule . . .' (1:26), and 'male and female he created them' as an explanation of 'So God created mankind in his own image' (1:27). We were made to be in human relationships as image-bearers of a personal God in trinitarian relationships.

Jesus, our Saviour, taught us that the greatest commandment is to love the Lord with all our heart, soul, mind and strength and the second greatest is to love our neighbour as ourselves (Luke 10:27). A godly life, one most clearly manifesting our likeness to God, is characterized by loving relationships with God and with other human beings. Michael Horton comments,

> To be created in God's image is to be called persons in
> communion. There was no moment when a human being

was actually a solitary, autonomous, unrelated entity; self-consciousness always included consciousness of one's relation to God, to each other and to one's place in the wider created environment.[6]

The qualities that constitute our image are therefore personal. They enable us to relate to God and other humans and to rule/work on the earth in the Lord's service. As Horton states, 'In sum, then, we may say that by the image of God . . . we mean the entire endowment of gifts and capacities that enable man to function as he should in his various relationships and callings.'[7]

We can make a shortlist of these godlike qualities. Usually in theology and medicine they are grouped into four categories: intellectual (reason/thinking/cognition), emotional (feeling), volitional (willing/desiring) and perceptual (sensing the world around us). Each of these categories is broad. There are different patterns of thinking and different kinds of emotion and so on. And they do not exist independently, but work together interacting and influencing one another.

Damaged image

The sin of Adam in Eden led God to curse his creation. He caused major changes throughout his universe. One was that he brought ageing, sickness and death into this world. But He did not remove our special image qualities. Human beings remain image-bearers (Genesis 9:6; James 3:9), able to think, feel and will, but now in a distorted and diminished way.

But the mentally ill are damaged in these qualities. They may be impaired intellectually (cognitively). They may lose their ability to learn and remember. Like my patient above, they hallucinate (perceiving things that are not really there) and become deluded (believing false things and losing contact with reality) and thus are unable to think rationally. Consequently, their ability to engage with other people and with God himself is damaged. And it can be hard for us to relate to them.

Everyone knows that Miriam is over-emotional. Not everyone knows why. Her bipolar disorder makes her emotions unstable. When she is well you wouldn't know this. But when she is ill she soars to heights of happiness and then crashes to withdrawn gloom. The emotional control component of her image has been loosened; it wobbles easily, sending her up and down. God himself has a full and perfect emotional range, with total self-control over his feelings and flawless responsiveness to us and his whole creation. But mental illnesses like Miriam's result in unstable and inappropriate emotional responses. They strike at this aspect of our image-ness.

Benji has autism. He doesn't understand personal cues. He struggles to communicate because he doesn't see the social signals. His use of language is odd and hard for others to comprehend. To be human is to be a communicating being, because God is. He uses language to speak to us in the Bible, and we use language as he does. But people on the autistic spectrum (that is, with severe autism or milder forms) have been damaged and disabled. They have lost some of our ability to use language and to understand social signals. This damage to their verbal and non-verbal communication leads to significant difficulties with relationships.

In these and other ways mental illness deranges our ability to function fully as human beings. While all sicknesses, at least to some extent, affect the whole of our being, mental illnesses strike directly at our image-ness. This is why they have always been so feared and stigmatized. The peculiar tragedy of mental illness is that it involves damage to the very properties of thinking, feeling, perceiving and acting that are central to humans as created in the likeness of God. Heart disease or osteoarthritis may be unpleasant, troublesome illnesses, but they don't directly affect these personal qualities that make humans special as God's image-bearers.

Work and mental illness

The immediate reason given for our image-ness is that we are to rule over all the earth under God (Genesis 1:26–28). This kingly role of acting for God on earth fits well with the meaning of image and likeness.[8] It is also wide-reaching. It includes scientific, technological and artistic enterprises. It has been called the 'cultural mandate', a phrase that captures its breadth. Since humans are spatially limited, then in order to rule the whole earth it was also necessary that we multiplied (1:28). More and more people would spread out to cover the earth and carry out this cultural mandate.

And so the two functions of rule and relationship are joined together. It is as people in relationships, in families and communities, that we express our kingly function. We live together inventing things, making things, enjoying exercising our skills. In the second creation account (Genesis 2:15) we are given a specific example of this when God commanded Adam to work and take care of the Garden of Eden.

The importance for us here is that work, creative and productive activity, is how human beings express our image. Such work is good for us. And work is not just what we get paid for. It is about using our unique skills and knowledge to express ourselves in God's service. We were created to be active in developing skills and learning about God's creation. This matures us.

So what happens when such activity is frustrated? We are damaged. Each stressful failure chips away at us and weakens us. We might fail in our work because of mental illness. Heather lost her job at Morrison's when she couldn't manage the checkout any more. She had always enjoyed the social interaction and the routine, but became embarrassed as she kept messing up. Later it became clear she had a dementia. This had caused her to lose the ability to use figures and read properly.

A stunning statement

Genesis 2:18 is amazing. The most amazing verse in the Bible? Perhaps not, for there is stiff competition. But here we read that it is not good for the man to be alone. Think about it. Surely in the Garden of Eden, in 'heaven on earth', Adam would be fulfilled? Walking and talking with his Creator, without any interference from sin or sickness would mean that Adam was blissfully happy, wouldn't it? Well, no, it wouldn't.

God himself tells us that it was not good. Or not completely good. God cannot pronounce his creation finished and very good because a lonely Adam was incomplete. Eve had to be created. She was needed to make him whole and enable him fully to express the image of God by having a relationship with another human person. This amazing verse teaches us the immense importance of human relationships.

Eve was made to complement Adam and provide him with the companionship of a fellow creature. No other living creature had been able to provide this companionship. In Genesis 2:19–20 we read that the other 'living creatures' (beasts of the field, livestock and birds) were brought to Adam. He named them, meaning he thought about their qualities and demonstrated his authority over them.

But when he studied them, not one was suitable to be his companion. He could not enjoy a personal relationship with any of them. So Eve, a fellow image-bearing human being, was made in order to meet this relational need. When Adam saw Eve, he rejoiced. At last here was 'bone of his bones and flesh of his flesh' (Genesis 2:23), a creature of the same stuff as himself. As Anthony Hoekema says, 'What is being said in this verse is that the human person is not an isolated being who is complete in himself or herself, but that he or she is a being who needs the fellowship of others, who is not complete apart from others.'[9]

Rule and relationship and mental illness

We are made to be creative and work under God. But in a fallen and cursed world work has become arduous. Most of the hardship and trials are minor. But if they persist, they can be significant stressors. A nasty criticism of your work performance or a personal insult in isolation has a different impact from nagging disparagement day in and day out. And such relentless stress can contribute to depression or an anxiety problem, at least in vulnerable individuals.

Recognizing that we are made to be in human relationships is crucial to understanding mental illness. These illnesses strike at those human qualities which enable us to form and mature such relationships, as well as damaging our kingly role in working for God (as happened to Heather above). Rule and relationship are the two key godlike functions given to us at creation. Each is affected by all types of sickness, but they are hit especially hard by mental illness.

Less frequently we experience more severe events, such as an accident, unemployment or bereavement. On their own these can tip us over into mental illness. Of course, such experiences do not lead to mental illnesses in most people most of the time. But for some they are important factors.

As unique as our fingerprints

We are not clones. We are made with personalities as individual as our irises or fingerprints. The qualities of one person fit alongside and enhance those of others. We carry one another's burdens and strengthen one another. In our relationships in the church we are family. We are made to find satisfaction in such relationships. And this has important implications for helping the mentally ill.

This reality of humans as relational creatures is why we see such a craving for satisfying relationships in everyone, but especially in those damaged souls who have been denied such blessings. Good relationships mature us and strengthen us and are indeed a great blessing. They can protect us against the impact of adverse experiences. But bad relationships harm us. They misshape us. They make us uncomfortable and fragile. They make us people who are vulnerable to mental illness.

Children reared in Christian homes should grow into the most stable and mature individuals, because they benefit from clear rules, stable circumstances and loving relationship, especially those who, by God's grace, come to faith at a young age. They are relaxed and at ease in relationships with other people of all kinds. They are stable emotionally and strong during crises. They are least vulnerable to mental illnesses. Of course, other homes that provide the same kind of environment will yield the same kind of benefits.

Such statements are not meant as a kind of apologetic. Nor do they imply that being brought up in a Christian family confers immunity to mental illness. Contributory factors, such as genetics and life experiences, can dominate and swamp the benefits of a Christian home. But a happy Christian home and a biblical upbringing do provide the best start for people. It reduces our vulnerability. Sadly, the opposite is true. We are aware of the damaging effects of a bad childhood, of the mentally harmful effects of an abusive home.

Jessica's marriage was close and happy. She ran the home well, and she and Tom did everything together. Until he walked out on her. Then she collapsed mentally. She refused to see her family, didn't look after herself and stopped attending church. Eventually she saw a psychiatrist and he learned about her appalling childhood. She had endured day after day of verbal abuse and relentless criticism. Politely, the message was 'You're useless and ugly.' Ostracized by her parents, she had no close friends, until she met Tom. And so his departure reawakened her feelings of misery and insecurity. Others have suffered much more and have been made more vulnerable as a result.

So are we all fragile creatures, ready to fall apart when troubles occur? Clearly not. We are incredibly robust. Nor is this to suggest that the Holy Spirit's sanctifying work, changing us daily to be ever more holy like Jesus Christ, is ineffective or unimportant. We can endure many adverse circumstances and many traumatic experiences without getting mentally ill. We are wonderfully made. Our bodies can heal well when injured without medical aid. Similarly, we are self-healing when wounded by events or relationships. Time, as we say, is a 'great healer'.

But the 'ordinary' support and practical help from family, friends and the church helps us to pull through the most distressing situations. It is meant to do so. We were created to be in such helpful relationships. But sometimes we cannot cope. Our personal resources are overwhelmed and we become mentally ill. And it is because we are different people with different susceptibilities and different degrees of endurance that some of us develop mental illnesses and some of us don't.

Damaged and further damaged

We are born with damaged souls along with damaged bodies. Such damage increases with our grim experiences in this cursed world. We are injured people who are afflicted by bereavements, natural disasters and accidents to friends and family. These events are outside our control but stress our weakened faculties.

Then there are all those afflictions that result from the sinful behaviour of others. We are afflicted when people lie to us and cheat us. We are stressed when we are insulted and scorned. We suffer when we are robbed and assaulted. Such stressors produce a stress response in us. They affect us body and soul. Mental stress changes hormones in the body (steroids) which make us prone to depression. And it changes the chemical dopamine in the brain, making us prone to psychosis and schizophrenia. Of course, such events do not simply affect the body. They make us sad or angry or fearful. They strain us, rendering us prone to mental illness.

Emotional reactions to stress are natural human responses. Remember that even a perfect man expressed strong emotions and struggled to bear such things. Jesus himself wept and was deeply affected by the horrible impact of sin and death on Lazarus and his family (John 11). At other times he struggled through with 'loud cries and tears' (Hebrews 5:7 ESV). He was a man of sorrows and acquainted with grief (see Isaiah 53:3).

If our sinless Saviour was deeply emotionally affected, then surely it is reasonable to expect sin-damaged people sometimes to become unable to bear the load. At times we cannot respond to such stressors with appropriate mental reactions like Jesus did. We break down. We are overwhelmed and develop a mental illness. Or do we suppose that we are mental supermen and women who can bear any load, withstand any pressure and come through smelling of roses?

Let's spell it out. Breakdown here does not involve personal sin. The depression, anxiety, worries and fears arise as a result of events and experiences external to the sufferer. They are not a result of their bad behaviour. Such events impact on a cursed and weakened soul. And the mental illness that arises from soul damage from psychological events (bereavement, insults, ostracism and so on) is analogous to bodily damage arising from physical disease.

The power of personal meaning

The essence of disease and illness is that it originates from events that happen to you. You don't control them; they control you. Damaged arteries stop enough blood getting to your heart and so you have a heart attack. You breathe in a flu virus and become sick. This also applies to psychological stressors and mental illness. Such events are solely mental or psychological in the sense that they involve no physical contact or transfer of any physical agent. But the absence of a physical component does not make them undamaging. It is the meaningfulness of unpleasant events that makes them powerful. The power of stressors lies in what they mean to us.[10]

When I heard on the news that an Islamist terrorist had killed eighty-six people in Nice by driving a cargo truck through a crowd, I was saddened. But not deeply. It had little personal meaning to me. However, if my children had been run over on the Promenade des Anglais, then I would have been heartbroken. My grief might have triggered a depressive illness.

Objectively this is the same event. Eighty-six people are killed. But my long and close relationships with my children means that the impact on me would be entirely different. The power of events to harm me psychologically lies in their impact on me. This isn't selfish or bad. It is simply a result of how we have been created.

As we saw earlier, we are made to have close relationships. And we will have others which are less close. The result is inevitably that some relationships have more power for harm than others. But the flipside is that some relationships have greater power to heal. Relationships are central to who we are and can be an immense blessing. We will see in later chapters how this applies in helping people with mental illness.

So adverse experiences and mental trauma are the soul/mind equivalent of bodily injury or infection. Just as bodily damage causes physical illness, so adverse experiences may produce mental illness. How do we categorize 'broken souls', people whose life experiences have damaged them and who develop mental illness as a result?

If the body was broken by heart disease or rheumatoid arthritis, we wouldn't have any difficulty in recognizing the vile influence of sin and the curse. And, crucially, we wouldn't blame the sufferer. These illnesses arise from disease processes acting on a weakened and ageing body. So why are 'broken souls' so often viewed differently? Why are people who develop mental illnesses due to psychological stressors frequently treated with scepticism? The answer is that mental illnesses are thought to be different. And, as we consider in the next chapter, because psychiatry has contributed to such confusion by wrongly defining mental illness.

Key chapter points

- The divine image is holistic (involves all our abilities, body and soul) and personal.
- Mental illness damages us holistically as persons.
- We were created to rule/work, which can either help us or harm us mentally.
- We were made for human relationships, and while these can be a source of stress, they are also a powerful means for helping people with mental illnesses.

3. WHAT IS MENTAL ILLNESS?

A few years ago I travelled with my family to the USA, and one of the highlights was visiting the Grand Canyon. While walking around the South Rim I was distracted from the magnificent views by a man coming towards us wearing a T-shirt bearing the words: 'I'm so old I remember when Pluto was a planet.' Do you remember the controversy about Pluto's planetary status? Was Pluto a planet after all?

It was striking because until then most of us had naively assumed that it was very easy to know what a planet was: it was a large spherical object that rotated around the sun (or, in other solar systems, around other stars). But of course it is not quite that simple. There are many other stony objects, such as asteroids, which circle round the sun and are not planets. But these are small. And planets need to be big. But how big? How large do you need to be to achieve planetary status? One view is that an object needs to be large enough for its gravity to force it into a spherical shape. Other experts disagree. Defining a planet turns out to be trickier than we had realized.

There are many other examples of difficulties with definitions. 'When is a land mass in the sea an island?' (Too small and it is simply a rock, too large and it becomes a continent.) 'What is a poem?' (How much imagery does it need? Does it have to rhyme? Does it show sufficient repetition?) Defining and categorizing things generally becomes tricky when you look more closely. Experts love to point out such complexities. Cynically, it appears that an expert is someone able to identify bamboozling problems in what the rest of us thought was straightforward.

So what is illness? And what is mental illness? As with planets, we all have a common-sense understanding. There are different definitions of mental illness and major disagreements in concepts. But we don't throw up our hands and say 'planets don't exist' just because there is no definition that all astronomers agree on. In the same way, the fact that definitions of mental illness differ doesn't mean mental illnesses are a false construct, a wrong-headed idea.

Does it matter how we define mental illness?

So what? You might wonder if it really makes any difference how we define mental illness. Well, it does. Ahmad has had problems in his marriage for some time. And now he has lost his job. He attends church infrequently and disappears quickly. You visit. He tells you he has depression. He shows you the antidepressants his GP has just prescribed and informs you he is seeing a counsellor. He is telling you this is not your business. This is medical. He has 'mental health problems' and this is nothing to do with the church, thanks very much.

But what is depression? Is he ill? A medical diagnosis is powerful. It (supposedly) identifies a problem and provides a solution. And that solution requires health service expertise, not any lowly church leader. You wouldn't try to help deal with heart disease or arthritis, would you? So why would you help with depression?

The definition of illness matters because it establishes legitimate spheres of power. This is turf war. Our society has allowed psychiatry to roll its tanks on to ministerial territory. If someone is ill, they need medical help. They still need input from family and the church, but not to deal with their medical illness. That is shut off. But what if Ahmad does not have depression and isn't ill after all?

Defining illness

We need to define mental illness. But it is important to place this in the larger category of illness in general. Disease involves damage to us, and this leads to illness, which is what we experience. Doctors look for diseases, medical causes that lead to people being ill or sick.

The Medline online dictionary (part of the prestigious National Institutes of Health (NIH) in the USA: http://www .nlm.nih.gov/medlineplus/mplusdictionary.html) defines illness as 'an unhealthy condition of *body or mind*'. We saw in chapter 1 the error of trying to restrict mental illness to the physical realm. If mental illness is genuine, then it should mean the same thing as any other kind of sickness and should be defined in the same way. And it is here by the NIH. It may involve body or mind.

Don't worry about the details that follow. Focus on the words in italics. The NIH defines disease as

> An *impairment* of the normal state of the living animal or
> plant body or one of its parts that interrupts or modifies the

performance of the vital functions, is typically manifested by distinguishing *signs and symptoms*, and is a *response to* environmental factors (as malnutrition, industrial hazards, or climate), to specific infective agents (as worms, bacteria, or viruses), to inherent defects of the organism (as genetic anomalies), or to combinations of these factors. (italics added for emphasis)

We note four elements in this definition:

1. Disease results from something that produces a response.
2. This something is an objective event (environmental factors, infective agents, etc.) outside the person's control.
3. Disease leads to signs and symptoms (which is what the person experiences as illness).
4. Disease produces clinically significant impairment in everyday functioning.

The element of response is important. It has two aspects: a triggering event ('something') and a change from healthy normality. This means that a disease results from something that happens to you. You were healthy, something happened and you responded by becoming ill. It required an objective cause. It was not your choice. This is the common-sense view of illness.

Just as a common-sense understanding of illness includes objective causation, so it also includes the idea of impairment. A sick person can't function normally. When we learn someone is ill, we understand this means he or she is not able to carry on living as usual. This is what we mean by 'clinically significant impairment in everyday functioning'.

Our definition of mental illness

A proper definition should follow the historical one above from NIH and include physical and psychological causes which trigger mental illness. **Our definition is that a mental illness is a behavioural syndrome (a collection of signs and symptoms) that results from a response to some objective cause or causes (external or internal), which may be physical or psychological, and these signs and symptoms produce clinically significant impairment in everyday functioning.**

To state that our concept of mental illness should include objective events is not to imply that we have to be able to prove such causes to allow someone to be diagnosed with an illness. Many mental illnesses remain mysterious. But this is also true of many other medical illnesses. The point is that in principle they are caused by some objective event or process. The concern here is that modern psychiatry's diagnostic manual (DSM[1]) does not in principle have a separable cause. For these the behaviour *is* the disorder.

Creation and inflation

DSM has created lots of new categories of 'mental health problems' (or 'mental disorders', as it calls them). This is because the common-sense requirement of causation has been removed. Thus, any behaviour individuals choose to engage in can be deemed a mental disorder.

And diagnoses are inflated when the need for impairment in everyday function is removed. In fairness, DSM does include the need for impairment. But when the diagnoses are let loose in the real world, this element is frequently ignored.

One of the most outspoken critics of *DSM-5* has been Allen Frances, who was the chair of *DSM-IV* and had a senior role in *DSM-III*. He summed up his concerns in his book *Saving Normal*.[2] Here he laments the loss of perspective on what illness is and thus the inflation of mental illnesses. He stridently criticizes the failure of *DSM-5* (repeating and extending the mistakes he now acknowledges with his own *DSM-IV*) to state more clearly what the boundaries should be for mental illness. The result is that the boundary between normality and illness is burst. So everyday distress becomes mental disorder. This is the turf where church leaders are equipped to help, but which psychiatry has claimed for medicine.

Creation: new mental disorders

Here is a question I use when teaching junior doctors: 'Which of the following is not an official mental disorder?' Motivational deficiency disorder, pyromania,[3] caffeine intoxication, exhibitionistic disorder or hoarding disorder? The correct answer is that the first one is not in DSM. So the rest are listed as mental disorders!

Motivational deficiency disorder was invented as part of a Finnish study investigating diagnoses in medicine.[4] It was ticked by a number of health professionals. If you read DSM (it is actually quite readable), you will find many 'mental disorders' akin to motivational deficiency disorder. It is quite easy to do what this study did and invent other similar sounding ones.

We could conceive of 'hijacking disorder' for disturbed individuals who take illegal control of aeroplanes or 'road rage disorder' for people who become angry and aggressive when frustrated by traffic. This arbitrary element to the DSM definition is one reason why it has been so widely criticized.[5] And a baleful consequence is that real and extremely debilitating illnesses, such as schizophrenia and dementia, are lumped together with absurd 'diagnoses' like caffeine intoxication and pyromania.

Some DSM diagnoses are variants of normal human behaviour, for example alcohol use disorder. Others are clearly patterns of bad behaviour, labelled as 'mental disorders', for example fetishistic disorder and paedophilic disorder. Why does DSM include such entities as mental disorders? Because DSM, along with modern psychiatry, has changed the definition of illness.

As we've seen, the DSM definition[6] does not require an objective cause. There is no need for an illness to be a response to something else. In DSM the behaviour itself is equivalent to the disorder. This is why any behaviour can be deemed a mental disorder if people don't like it. We see this with diagnoses such as paedophilia or caffeine intoxication. And this is why the 'illness' word is shunned in DSM and psychiatry today. Instead, we have the more flexible 'disorder'. This is not accidental. It is a deliberate departure from the above medical definition and historical understanding of disease and illness.[7]

So someone who chooses to repeatedly set fires because they enjoy it can be diagnosed with 'pyromania'. Someone who drinks lots of alcohol and becomes intoxicated and aggressive can be diagnosed with 'alchohol intoxication'. These DSM mental disorders, like many others, are simply bad[8] behaviours. Bad behaviour is not illness. Sin is not sickness.[9]

Surely this is another reason why the definition of mental illness matters, isn't it? Once we allow sinful behaviour to be classified as illness, then we allow people to deny responsibility for such behaviour. Or at least to minimize it. Who likes blaming a sick person for behaving badly? We feel for them and want to help them. We will focus on this important issue in chapter 6 where we think about how we balance the compassion we feel for the sick with their responsibility for their behaviour.

Real-world psychiatry

It is important to clarify that psychiatrists in the UK don't go around diagnosing caffeine intoxication and tobacco use disorder. In everyday practice DSM is hardly used at all. So why the fuss? Partly because DSM diagnoses are what junior doctor psychiatrists are taught to use (although when I teach diagnosis, they hear a critical view of DSM!). And even when we abandon them as consultants, our thinking is still heavily shaped by them. We tend to overdiagnose, following the artificial creation and inflation of DSM some of the way.

And most research studies in psychiatry use DSM. So when choosing treatments we are again pushed along DSM lines of thinking. Also DSM greatly helps the expansion of psychiatry into the domain of struggling with life's difficulties. It medicalizes and legitimizes this medical land grab. So people like Ahmad get dealt with by the health service instead of being helped by church and family.

Inflation: no bright line between normality and mental illness

Ahmad was wrongly given a diagnosis of depression. Depression is a genuine illness, not a DSM creation. But one which has been hugely inflated to include the kind of life struggles Ahmad was experiencing. Normal reactions to stressful circumstances are allowable as mental disorders.

Thus, here there are potential objective psychological causes of illness. Ahmad had experienced stressful circumstances. But we all have such experiences, in much the same way as we all have bodily aches and pains. So when does someone actually become ill?

The answer is that we become ill when we are impaired in our everyday living: in the words of our definition, when we have 'clinically significant impairment'. This is a medical judgment call, the kind doctors make daily when determining someone is sick. But it requires a determination to distinguish a normal stress response from illness. DSM discourages us from identifying normal distress.

Sociologist Owen Whooley states,

> The symptoms-based diagnostic categories of the DSM fail to situate symptoms in the life experiences of an individual and thus provide no context that might distinguish normal distress in life from genuinely pathological conditions that indicate underlying mental illness . . . This leads . . . to inflated rates of mental disorders in community.[10]

In real-world clinical work psychiatrists do not carry out the kind of unthinking approach that DSM implies. We do think about the person. We want to understand why this unique individual has reacted to that event in this way. We all recognize that Gareth is an anxious lad, a worrier, while Sam is relaxed. In the months approaching college exams Gareth becomes tense and edgy, not sleeping properly and worrying about how he would do. Sam remains laid-back. To diagnose Gareth with an anxiety disorder is legitimate according to DSM. But this would be absurd, wouldn't it?

Michelle is labile emotionally, that is, prone to respond somewhat excessively to experiences. If she is successful in her exams, she will be euphoric, bounding around like a puppy dog. But if she fails she will be in despair. Such transient reactions are typical of Michelle and expected. They are not abnormal. Yet by DSM she could be diagnosed as having a hypomanic episode or even bipolar disorder if she had had previous 'episodes'. Hopefully in the real world such reactions would be recognized as being characteristic of Michelle as a person. But they aren't always. And the tendency is to encourage such normal reactions to be diagnosed as mental disorders. And thus to imply to church leaders that they are not our business.

Medicalization of society

The rest of medicine faces the same dilemma as psychiatry in trying to determine where the boundary between sickness and health lies. There is no bright line, but a fuzzy and indistinct one on a continuum between health and sickness. When someone has moderate or severe illness, whether heart disease or schizophrenia, it is easy to say they are ill. But when it is mild and near the fuzzy line, it is difficult.

Take hypertension (high blood pressure). Recent guidelines lowered the blood pressure threshold so that mild hypertension could be diagnosed at a systolic blood pressure of only 140mmHg. Suddenly an astonishing 22% of the world's adult population were caught in the hypertensive net![11] Determining correct thresholds is tricky. But changing thresholds has converted vast numbers of symptom-free people into patients on treatment.

Many symptoms of sickness can also be everyday experiences unrelated to sickness, such as tiredness/fatigue, shortness of breath, poor sleep, pains, sadness and poor concentration. Usually we live with these without thinking we are ill. When do we become worried? Generally, when the symptoms persist and/or become severe enough to affect our daily lives. This is what lies behind the concept of clinically significant impairment. Roughly, it is clinically significant when the doctor agrees with the patient's own assessment that the symptoms are having an important impact on his or her everyday life.

Inflation in psychiatry

So today large numbers of people with normal distress have been converted into people with mental illnesses. The American National Comorbidity Study Replication (NCS-R: http://www.hcp.med.harvard.edu/ncs/) conducted a face-to-face household survey between February 2001 and April 2003 applying *DSM-IV* criteria. They reported that the incidence, in American adults, of mood disorders over a lifetime is 20.8%, and for anxiety disorders, 28.8%. They also reported that, over a lifetime, 57.4% will have at least one mental disorder. These figures are said to be an underestimate (!) because they did not survey some major mental illnesses, such as schizophrenia and dementia. And of course they did not include children.

In England, you may be pleased to learn, things are much better. The Adult Psychiatric Morbidity Survey (APMS) (http://www.hscic.gov.uk/pubs/psychiatricmorbidity07) assessed psychiatric disorders in English households in 2007 and reported that 'only' 23% of adults had at least one mental disorder. While this survey was more comprehensive, it still did not include some categories, such as dementia.

Determining clinical significance

How much depression does someone have to experience following some stress to be diagnosed as having a depressive illness? How anxious do you need to be when under pressure at work to have an anxiety illness? If someone affected by a psychological stressor, such as bereavement, is coping at work and functioning as usual at home and at church, he or she does not have clinically significant distress and is not ill. But if that person becomes sad and withdrawn after such a stressful experience, and can't manage commitments at home and work, then he or she could be diagnosed with depression.

Is this not a bit subjective? Yes. Unavoidably. It is a personal judgment. Diagnosis is not made by a machine using objective and scientifically proven criteria. There is no bright line dividing normal from abnormal. We considered the problems of definitions at the beginning of this chapter. There is no objective criterion for how big an object circulating the sun has to be in order to be a planet. And there is no objective criterion for how high a sugar level has to be for a diabetes diagnosis to occur or how high blood pressure has to be for hypertension to be diagnosed.

But subjective is not random. Decisions are made for clinical reasons built (in theory at least) on scientific evidence. In their discussion of the definition of mental illness, Stein and colleagues comment that no definition precisely specifies the boundaries of mental illness.[12] But they also observe that this is true for all illnesses: 'We would add that no definition of which we are aware perfectly specifies precise boundaries for the concept of non-psychiatric medical disorder either.'[13]

People behaving strangely

Some years ago I was sitting in a meeting at Newcastle University listening to a couple of case presentations[14] intended for instruction in complex aspects of an illness. But that day it was about a tricky legal issue and so attracted a wider audience. I was sitting next to a senior professor in neuro-science who leaned over at the end and whispered, 'You psychiatrists ought to get out more. He wasn't mentally ill, just wacky . . . you should know that . . . you get all sorts of wacky people in church.' I agreed with him. I know he didn't mean that all Christians are wacky. But we do get a lot of odd people in our churches. Society is full of people whose behaviour I find peculiar. But they are not mentally ill, most of them anyway.

Our personality is unique. We have our very own pattern of acting and interacting, of thinking and feeling and per-ceiving the world. We all know the great range and variety of people's personalities, and we rejoice in this wonderful aspect of God's creation. Mary is melancholic and naturally gloomy. Thus low mood and pessimistic thinking are typical of her (the gloomy Eeyore was her favourite character in the Winnie the Pooh books!). In someone else, her behaviour, especially when she has problems at home, might raise concern about depression. But not when we know Mary well.

Bruce has always been a bit sensitive to criticism. So sus-piciousness and 'paranoid behaviour' in him is normal. But in someone else it might suggest possible schizophrenia. Determining what is normal for one person and what is a change driven by illness can be difficult. When we draw the boundary between normality and mental illness, we need to be careful we don't sweep into the illness category people whose lifestyles and beliefs and behaviour are not mainstream.

Diagnosis is not always difficult

Most of the time diagnosis is straightforward, at least for an experienced doctor. In many cases it is easy for everyone. If you go to an inpatient psychiatric unit, you will find many suffering people whose illness is obvious. You don't need to be a doctor, let alone a psychiatrist, to see that someone with acute psychotic depression is ill.

This is true generally in medicine. When someone has a classical stroke (e.g. they have right-sided paralysis and slurred speech), or acute asthma (with shortness of breath and prominent wheezing), then the diagnosis is not difficult. But many people with stroke present with vague symptoms. Many with asthma have a repeated cough and subtle breathing problems only with exercise. Mild illnesses are always more difficult to identify in medicine because they are near the fuzzy boundary with normality.

We might prefer everything to be neat and tidy. It would be great if diagnosis was always easy (you wouldn't need doctors!), but often it isn't. However, we should put this in perspective. Those near the blurred line are also those who are less sick. Consequently, they have much less to gain from medical treatment. And those on the normal side have nothing at all to gain, and much to lose. We return again to the 'does it matter?' question.

It matters because you can help

It is not good to be alone. We saw earlier that we are created to be in relationships. And these relationships matter. They are important for restoring troubled souls. People in churches are a powerful source of help to the needy. People like Ahmad, wrongly diagnosed with depression, need the help of ministers and other Christians. Shutting them off behind a greatly expanded diagnostic fence and medicalizing their problems is unhelpful.

Psychiatric treatments don't work for such people. They need the support and care of brothers and sisters in Christ. It is well known that diagnoses empower doctors. But many psychiatric diagnoses disempower ministers and churches. They block us out from providing the pastoral care that distressed normal people need. People like Ahmad can be supported and treated by their family and the church. We will consider this later in chapters 8 and 9, where we will also see how church leaders are equipped to provide help to those with mental illnesses too. But first, we need to understand some of the reasons why people become mentally ill.

Key chapter points

- Modern psychiatry has redefined mental illness into mental disorder, which in the public domain has expanded to 'mental health problems'.
- True illness results from an objective cause (something happens to you to make you ill).
- Bad behaviours are now called mental disorders and mental health problems.
- Normal reactions to life's difficulties are frequently diagnosed as mental disorders.
- Such diagnoses make it difficult for churches to help people.

4. FREUD AND THE UNCONSCIOUS

I have no beard. Nor a moustache. And I've never asked a patient to lie on a couch. Yet even today the media image of the archetypal psychiatrist is of a bearded man sitting in a chair behind a patient who is reclining on a couch. This Freudian image is wrong in every way. Psychiatrists don't do psychoanalysis. We are doctors who do clinical interviews. Our patients sit on chairs as we do. We rarely have beards. Most of us are women after all! And Freud wasn't even a psychiatrist; he was a neurologist.

But such was the influence of Freud on twentieth-century Western culture that, although this view of the psychiatrist is riddled with errors, it remains a potent myth. More importantly, not only is this image of Freud in error, but most Freudian teaching is error too. It has been weighed in the scientific balance and found wanting. However, Freud and those who followed him did make the reality and the importance of the unconscious mind widely known. And on this at least he agreed with the Bible.

The Bible and the unconscious

We use 'unconscious'[1] here to refer to that mental activity which is not within conscious awareness. Obvious, I hope. And such activity is continuous and normal. Human beings are unique creatures because we can think not only about others but also about ourselves. Often when thinking, we become aware of the difficulty in interpreting and weighing our inner mental processes. As the prophet Jeremiah declared, 'The heart is deceitful above all things, and beyond cure. Who can understand it?' (17:9). Our minds are immensely complex and have vast hidden depths.

As usual in the Bible, 'heart' here refers to that thinking, feeling and willing aspect of our inner being. In our hearts we are sin-afflicted. We cannot correctly evaluate the thoughts and attitudes of our own hearts. We deceive ourselves inwardly about the motivation for our behaviour. We struggle to determine whether we have done good or ill. Yet Jeremiah's great consolation was that although we cannot see into the depths of our being, the Lord can. Similarly, Solomon prayed to the Lord, 'Deal with everyone according to all they do, since you know their hearts (for you alone know every human heart)' (1 Kings 8:39). We have hidden depths, which only the Lord can penetrate.

Our autopilot

Most of our mental activity occurs outside our conscious awareness, in the subconscious or unconscious. Typing this, my fingers move and my eyes read without my being aware of their activity, until, like now, I focus upon such matters. Every day we do things unconsciously, on 'autopilot'. We get out of bed, wash and dress, have breakfast and head off to work, college or school. We do not think, as we once did as children, 'I need to put my right leg in this trouser leg and my left leg in that one and then pull up my trousers.' We have learned the behaviour so thoroughly that it is automatic. Psychologists call this overlearned behaviour.

A good example of more complex unconscious behaviour is driving. I drive off in the morning following my usual route to my office at the hospital. For some of the time, often most of it, I am absorbed in thoughts about a meeting I'm chairing later in the day. Or thinking about a difficult clinic. Or I'm reflecting on the Bible teaching yesterday. But I am not thinking about the driving. This is a highly complex activity, yet one I regularly do without conscious mental effort. I'm on autopilot.

Once upon a time I learned to drive. I had to think consciously about the clutch pedal and engaging the gear and looking in my mirror and so on. But through endless practice I've embedded such behaviours in my unconscious. And this is true for much else too, isn't it? We repeat certain actions or activities so often that we not only learn them, but we overlearn them. They become automatic or habitual. They become embedded in the unconscious. We overlearn a whole range of daily habits (shaving, washing, dressing, eating, drinking, walking, cycling and so on).

A God of habit

We learn and acquire habits because we are made in the image of a God who is a God of habit. Every morning the sun rises and every evening it sets because the Lord is working day after day in the same way in his universe. He has promised that the regularity of the days and seasons will continue until the end of this created order (Genesis 8:22). We tend to describe their movements as working by the laws of science, but such laws are really God's habitual way of running his universe, aren't they? I am not suggesting that God does these things unconsciously. We cannot understand the mind of the Lord because he is so vastly greater than we are (Job 38 – 41; Isaiah 40). But the point is that he works in regular and predictable ways in so much of what he does in the universe. He is a God of habit, and we are created in his image so will naturally also be creatures of habit.

Drive like a Christian

When driving, I've sometimes seen bumper stickers or window stickers requesting me to 'drive like a Christian'. What does this mean? Can moral behaviour be unconscious too? We may be able to accept such humdrum matters as washing and dressing as unconscious. But is this true also when I obey God? Is righteousness often unconscious? The above reflections on the unconscious may be uncontentious. But once we move to moral behaviour, you may become uncomfortable.

But this is a false distinction, isn't it? There is nothing in the Bible to suggest any difference between moral behaviour and other behaviour. Paul tells the Corinthians, 'Whether you eat or drink, or whatever you do, do it all for the glory of God' (1 Corinthians 10:31). All our behaviour is done before God and should please him. In this sense it is all moral. Paul has been saying that eating meat sacrificed to idols is fine since it is only meat. It is a part of God's good creation and is to be enjoyed. But the manner in which you eat it may be right or wrong. You may selfishly not think about the effect this behaviour will have on weak (less well-taught) Christians. They do not know that idols are nothings, and so they become drawn into idolatrous behaviour. Some behaviour (like worshipping idols) is just wrong. It is unlawful, that is to say, sin (1 John 3:4). Any (lawful) behaviour is morally good when we do it by faith in Christ to glorify God. Or it can be made bad because of our selfish attitudes or lack of faith.

So when driving on autopilot, perhaps the way in which I've learned to drive has ingrained bad behaviour? On my way to the hospital I might rudely cut in suddenly in front of someone. I selfishly assert my right to the road over theirs. This may be my habitual way of driving. But it is wrong. You might say, 'It is unconscious and so how can you be at fault?' But there is no Scripture which teaches a 'get-out clause' for unconscious behaviour, is there? I may have done it without thinking, unconsciously. But I did it. It is therefore my fault, my sin.

Excusing sin

I think that much, perhaps all, of the antipathy among Christians to the concept of the unconscious is that it has been used to excuse sin. I remember attending an ordination service and queuing for some (pretty awful) tea and biscuits when suddenly I became aware of an outburst from the woman in front of me. Violet was rudely rebuking this young innocent in no uncertain terms. It was embarrassing. And it was horrible and wicked. I commented to Violet's minister on her rudeness and how upset the young woman on the receiving end was. 'Oh, don't worry about Violet,' he chuckled. 'That is just her habit; she is always like that.' This is far from the only occasion when I've seen habitual and unconscious behaviour like that excused. You don't need a clear concept of the unconscious to use it to excuse sin.

'It wasn't my fault because it is just my (or his or her) habit' is a wrong conclusion to draw. It has no biblical warrant.

Significantly, in the above example from 1 Corinthians 10:31, it is the ordinary, and usually unconscious, behaviours of eating and drinking that Paul singles out as conduct that can be done sinfully or to the glory of God. Whether we act consciously or unconsciously, and whether our acts are special or routine, we should be aiming to bring praise to God in them all.

Mind your Ps and Qs

How do we develop our unconscious behaviours? I've stated above that routine behaviours are repeated so often that they become what psychologists call 'overlearned'. We develop ingrained behaviours of varying levels of complexity. We call them 'habits'. They are patterns laid down in our unconscious. These habitual behaviours may be good or bad.

Making such behaviour ingrained in our children is part of what being a good parent involves. Proverbs 22:6 teaches us: 'Start children off on the way they should go, and even when they are old they will not turn from it.' We aim to instil sound conduct in our children when they are young and most malleable and are still forming their behaviours. We teach them to say 'please' and 'thank you' so that such courtesy becomes habitual and enables them to be unconsciously polite in social situations. We train them in a myriad of ways by our explicit teaching, by our discipline and by our example. We model kind practices, like visiting the sick or lonely, and giving lifts to the elderly and infirm.

We want such loving behaviour to become part of their developing character. Then, when they grow up, much of their kind and generous behaviour is unconscious. They phone someone who is ill to check how he or she is doing and learn this person would like to come to church. Instantly they suggest they could provide a lift. Sometimes such behaviour is consciously thought through, and sometimes it is unconscious, a habit. But whether it is conscious or unconscious, it still is an aspect of Christian love, of morally good behaviour. Consistent biblical training will assist in the development of a balanced and mature person.

Teaching good habits is difficult because our children are born sinners. They tend towards bad habits. And we, their role models, are flawed ourselves. Thus Proverbs 22:15 warns us that 'Folly is bound up in the heart of a child, but the rod of discipline will drive it far away.' Most of the time children need teaching, example and loving guidance. But sometimes parental love also necessitates physical discipline.

Christian parents strive by example and teaching to embed good habits. So you meet a young boy who opens the door for you, smiles and welcomes you to his home, and on leaving you give him a small gift, to which he responds instinctively by saying 'thank you'. This kind and polite behaviour has been drilled into him. He has developed these good habits. Funnily, I've heard people claim that such behaviour doesn't count morally just because it is habitual. But when children are surly and rude by habit, as a result of poor upbringing and example, then their thanklessness is typically condemned. We are so inconsistent.

Sadly, this opposite kind of parenting, bad parenting, is all too common. Too many children experience abusive behaviour that is damaging, resulting in disintegrated, unstable and emotionally volatile people. You may meet a young boy who is surly, avoids eye contact and, when irritated, becomes angry and swears. And he is to blame for this bad behaviour, isn't he? Again it is easy to see that such habits have been learned. They have also become ingrained through his experience. In his case this folly, this foolish and wicked pattern of behaviour, has not been driven out by discipline. And instead, it has been taught and modelled by angry and rude parents. In biblical terms, such failure indicates a lack of love: Proverbs 13:24, for instance, tells us, 'Whoever spares the rod hates their children, but the one who loves their children is careful to discipline them.' Our heavenly Father disciplines us, so we should imitate him in disciplining our children. True love can involve painful words and the infliction of physical pain, as exemplified by God in his dealings with us (Hebrews 12:5–11).

Old dogs can learn new tricks

It is clear that many habits, for better or worse, are laid down in childhood. But we continue to learn and embed habits as adults. For example, we don't begin to learn to drive until we are adults, and yet driving habits can become deeply ingrained. Jesus worked with his closest twelve disciples and with a much larger band of followers to train them as adults. His whole approach demonstrates that learning and maturing behaviour continue throughout life. Writing to the Ephesians (4:11–13), Paul says that God has given us different proclaimers of the truth (apostles, prophets, evangelists, pastor-teachers), who by their teaching build up Christians in unity and maturity so we all become increasingly Christlike. And he goes on (4:25ff.) to teach how in turn all believers should be proclaiming truth to their brothers and sisters in Christ. All our inter-actions should work together with the formal truth-tellers to shape our behaviour for good.

Sometimes we are told that adults are old dogs who can't learn new tricks. But if adults could not change, then why would Paul bother to teach this? Why would Jesus have spent so long training his disciples? We make progress by getting rid of bad habits and refining good ones. As we learn, we reflect on Bible teaching and make a conscious effort to become like Jesus. Chris was converted to faith in Christ from a world of heavy drinking. He had a lot to change, a lot of hard work to do. Should he drink at all? Did he have the self-discipline to drink within limits? Could he go near places where alcohol was consumed, knowing that its potent smell might overwhelm him? He had his daily routines and weekly patterns to change. He knew that habits of a lifetime needed to be broken and new ones needed to be rebuilt. He had to learn to relate to workmates, friends and family in new ways. A whole range of unhelpful and bad habitual behaviours had to be broken down and replaced with new routines and patterns that enabled him to live a very different Christlike life.

Give me the child and I'll give you the man

Such sanctification involves destroying bad unconscious habits, crucifying these aspects of our old self and replacing them with godly unconscious behaviours (initially with much conscious effort). This can be especially difficult when the behaviour is habitual from childhood. We want to train good habits into our children which cannot be removed later in life (Proverbs 22:6). But by the same token bad habits are also deeply embedded and difficult to shift.

The Jesuits, possibly Ignatius Loyola, are said to have coined the phrase: 'Give me a child until he is seven and I'll give you the man.' Whatever its original source, this captures the deeply ingrained nature of behaviours and character established in childhood. I know a Christian minister who swears. Although I've never heard him do so, he tells me he still struggles with this habit decades after his conversion. His upbringing formed the habit of swearing aloud at every kind of irritation and frustration. He continues to work day by day against this ingrained bad habit.

Some people have had much more difficult childhood experiences, which have left deep scars. Abuse in its different forms is, sadly, usually a repeated experience for many children and leads to ingrained maladaptive behaviours. A lack of trust in other people, especially authority figures, fragile confidence, poor self-esteem and emotional instability result from difficult and abusive experiences. These make it difficult for them in later life to form and sustain strong and nurturing relationships, also leading to problems in study and work.

Those key elements, demonstrating our divine image which we considered in chapter 2 (ruling and relating), are expressed badly because they have been damaged. These image qualities are misshaped by grim experiences. Such people are vulnerable to various mental illnesses. We will think about the stress-vulnerability model of mental illness in the next chapter. Here we simply note that unconscious aspects of our personality related to earlier experiences can leave people prone to such illnesses. And in terms of our definition of mental illness, these psychological experiences are objective factors which impact on us and make us prone to mental illnesses.

Freud and Freudianism

Since the Bible teaches the existence and influence of the unconscious, it is not surprising that people down the ages have recognized and sought to understand it. Although it is often thought that Sigmund Freud discovered the unconscious, this is not so. Freud was simply one man in a long line who theorized about the impact of unconscious processes on human behaviour. Henri Ellenberger, in his magisterial work

The Discovery of the Unconscious,[2] traces the changes in people's interpretation of the unconscious. He begins in ancient societies, moves through use of magnetism, then hypnotism and down to modern Freudian interpretations.[3]

So Freud didn't discover the unconscious, but he was an expert publicist. He made famous not just the reality of the unconscious mind but a complex framework of proposed unconscious mental mechanisms. Ellenberger discusses why Freud achieved such fame. His French contemporary Pierre Janet developed many of the same ideas but is unknown today. He concludes that Freud was a hard-working man with a powerful personality, who was lucky in his timing because his theories fitted the early twentieth-century zeitgeist.

Freud attempted to develop techniques (such as free association and dream analysis) to probe the unconscious. He also proposed models (which changed over time) of how the unconscious is supposed to work. Other Freudians proposed different models. They argued and disintegrated into a variety of warring factions. But all their models of the unconscious are untestable and hence unscientific (see below). They also conflict with biblical teaching (see further below). As Ellenberger observes, different Freudians have proposed different models that are contradictory and cannot be harmonized, which shows the precarious nature of this approach.[4]

Contrary to popular understanding, Freudianism has always been a minority position in psychiatry. He had the largest impact in the USA (ironic, since Freud famously hated America). And since the USA came to dominate twentieth-century popular culture, this was one way he got lucky. In other parts of the world, such as Germany and the UK, Freud never made a large impact at all. The highly influential German psychiatrist Karl Jaspers wrote in 1957,

'Freud's influence was limited to small circles. Psychological approaches were regarded to be subjective and futile, not scientific.'[5]

Most psychiatrists continued to adhere to a 'medical model'. The apparent success of Freudianism in psychiatry was always a mirage produced because of its wider cultural influence, particularly on the arts and humanities. Attempts to interpret films, dramas, plays and so on in Freudian terms continue today. But within psychiatry Freudian thinking has almost totally disappeared.

Freudianism: science or religion?

The details of Freud's theories, and of those who followed him, are beyond the scope of this work. They proposed models of different interacting forces in the unconscious, which are supposed to emerge as symptoms and behaviours. These forces are assumed to operate at a deeper level than the more subconscious level of overlearned behaviours above. These problems, then, may be identified as mental illnesses. Such features, buried deeply, are alleged to disguise their unconscious origin and thus to require psychotherapeutic skill to unmask them. The Freudian psychoanalyst probes to identify the real, underlying unconscious problems that are supposed to have generated these symptoms.

Historian Andrew Scull comments, 'Freud had stitched together psychoanalysis, as both theory and practice, on the foundation of his own hysterical breakdown, and the experience of ministering to a handful of hysterical women in the 1890s.'[6] Formulating a theory of human behaviour on the basis of observations made on oneself and a few late nineteenth-century bourgeois Viennese women is not how good science is done.

Freudianism has long been criticized as not proper science at all. It has always had a religious feel to it because it aims at life improvement, rather than treatment of illness. Since its inception many doctors have regarded it as mythological or religious, rather than scientific. In 1896, when Freud gave one of his early public lectures at the Society of Psychiatry and Neurology in Vienna, Richard von Krafft-Ebing, the eminent psychiatrist chairing, commented that his theory sounded like a fairy tale.[7] Summarizing the situation in 1970, Ellenberger wrote,

> The validity of psychoanalytic concepts is still questioned by many psychologists and epistemologists . . . many Freudians view psychoanalysis as a discipline that stands outside the field of experimental science and more akin to history, philosophy, linguistics, or as a variety of hermeneutics.[8]

How Einstein undid Freud

Freudianism was in his sights when philosopher of science Karl Popper developed his falsifiability test for scientific theories. Like Freud, he lived in early twentieth-century Vienna. Popper pondered the theories of Marx, Freud, Adler and Einstein. Each claimed to be scientific, but he felt uneasy about the first three. His thinking was clarified when Einstein's general theory of relativity was tested in 1919 during a solar eclipse. The outcome provided evidence confirming that the gravitational pull of the sun did indeed bend the path of light from distant stars, as predicted by Einstein. He realized that if the light had not been bent by the sun, then Einstein's theory would have been proven false. But he then saw that for the other three theories there was no conceivable experiment that could falsify them: 'The two psycho-analytic theories [of

Freud and Adler] were in a different class. They were simply non-testable, irrefutable. There was no conceivable human behaviour which could contradict them.'[9]

A true scientific theory has to be testable. You need to be able to carry out experiments to check it out. And although it may feel paradoxical, these tests also need to be able to show it is wrong. If you can't falsify it, it isn't science. Myths are ways of explaining phenomena, but their explanations are not scientific because there is no way they can be falsified. Freudianism is such a myth. An attempt to explain our behaviour based on hypothetical invisible and unmeasurable unconscious forces. The interactions of these forces can, like all good mythological systems, be used to 'explain' any behaviour whatsoever. But they can't be tested. Popper stated that 'for Freud's epic of the Ego, the Super-ego and the Id, no substantially stronger claim to scientific status can be made for it than for Homer's collected stories from Olympus'.[10]

Does it help?

So Freudianism is unscientific. But perhaps it helps people? It doesn't. In the 1980s the absence of evidence for any benefit from Freudian therapy was revealed during a court case in the USA.[11] Dr Osheroff, a physician, became ill with depression. In January 1979 he was admitted to Chestnut Lodge private hospital in Maryland, one of the major psychiatric institutions in the USA and a bastion of psychotherapy.

Here Dr Osheroff was treated with intensive individual psychotherapy four times a week, but was not given any anti-depressants. He and his family asked for these drugs. But they were told they would interfere with the psychotherapy. After seven months at Chestnut Lodge he had lost forty pounds in weight, suffered severe insomnia and had such severe agitation that his feet became blistered and required medical treatment. His family managed to get him transferred to Silver Hill Foundation in Connecticut. Here he was prescribed anti-depressants and antipsychotics for his psychotic depression. He recovered fully within three months and was able to return to his medical practice. In 1982 Dr Osheroff sued Chestnut Lodge for malpractice.

The doctors at Chestnut Lodge based their treatment approach on their Freudian theory of Dr Osheroff's condition. But in court they had to admit there was no evidence from clinical trials to support this approach in depression. The only evidence for this type of psychotherapy at the time was in schizophrenia, where two trials had shown that it did not produce any benefits for patients. Several psychiatrists at the hearing declared that there was substantial evidence from randomized controlled clinical trials (the gold standard for evidence in medicine) for the benefits of antidepressants. But there was no such evidence for this psychotherapy. Consequently, Dr Osheroff won substantial damages from the arbitration panel. Chestnut Lodge, after appeal, finally chose to settle out of court in 1987. They didn't want to risk a final judicial ruling against psychotherapy. Not the approach of people confident of their position.

It is important to note that concerns about the lack of evidence for benefits from Freudian psychotherapy in the Osheroff case and related literature should not tar all types of psychotherapy as ineffective. As we will see, other psycho-therapies, especially cognitive-behavioural therapy, have good evidence demonstrating benefits.

So Freudianism is myth and not science. And it doesn't work. Its theories and models of mental illness have been weighed in the balance and found wanting. When a therapist has probed away, fathoming the unconscious of the client (assuming that this is actually what is happening), the therapist will still only know a fraction of what is there. And they have this in incoherent fragments. So therapists need their theoretical models to try to make sense of this data. But these models are broken. Their theories have failed the acid test of science.

So what does the Bible teach on interpreting the unconscious?

Help from Donald Rumsfeld

Former US Secretary of Defence Donald Rumsfeld famously declared about potential terrorists and their threats, 'There are known knowns. These are things we know that we know. There are known unknowns. That is to say, there are things that we know we don't know. But there are also unknown unknowns. There are things we don't know we don't know.' To modify this with respect to our sinful behaviour, we know sometimes when we've done wrong: these are our known knowns. Sometimes we don't recognize our wrongs: we are blind to them and need someone to point them out. These are our unknowns, which are known to others. Then there are those sins hidden so deeply that they are unknown both to us and to others. These unknown unknowns are known only to God.

We can't hope to understand the complex hidden depths of our minds. But we can acknowledge that sometimes other people see things that we don't see about ourselves. They know what is unknown to us. They can point out some of our failings to us. And if they know us well, they can see patterns of behaviour that we don't. And they can interpret (or guess, if you prefer) why we might be behaving as we do.

Dawn lived with stigma all her childhood. She was an illegitimate child born and raised in Ireland. Her Catholic parents refused the offered abortion but shunned her. As did everyone else. She was never kissed or cuddled. She was given all the dirty jobs to do at home. But then she met some Christians. People who were kind to her and truly wanted to know her. She attended church, heard the gospel and was converted to lasting faith in Christ. And she also met Tony. He learned about her grim life but still loved her. He learned more and more examples of the cold cruelty of her childhood. Her special blessing was that Tony was also a psychiatric nurse. He could see how her past would express itself in aloofness and detachment. He understood why she didn't like social events at church and he worked patiently with her. And when she got post-natal depression with their first child, he knew why this expressed itself in such strongly detached, isolating and mute behaviour. He could understand what she struggled to understand about herself. With Tony able to provide more than empathic support, and with anti-depressants, Dawn recovered. And continues to recover today.

Although the Bible teaches the existence and influence of the unconscious mind, it never provides any technique or model to help us to understand and explore the unconscious. Perhaps it even pushes in the opposite direction, for we read, 'The heart is deceitful above all things and beyond cure' (Jeremiah 17:9). We are told that only the Lord can know its confusing contents. In Psalm 19:12 the psalmist laments that he cannot know himself and his hidden errors. Paul declared that the Lord will expose his hidden depths, those unconscious thoughts and desires which drove him. He won't claim he is innocent of sin even when he isn't consciously aware of any sins. He knows he can sin unconsciously (1 Corinthians 4:1–5). These texts suggest that men like David and Paul, aware of the reality of hidden sins lurking in the depths of their hearts, did examine themselves to try to discern the potential sinfulness of their behaviour. But they realized they could not conduct a thorough self-investigation. They knew that finally they could only throw up their hands in failure and cast themselves on the mercy of the Lord (see Psalm 139:23–24).

Missing the obvious?

Perhaps you think I am overanalysing things? Am I not missing the obvious? Bad experiences are stressful and we know it. We are conscious, too well aware sometimes, that nasty events in the past affect our mind and precipitate emotional turmoil and worries. We don't need to rack our brains thinking through the impact of these on us through the unconscious mind, do we? I sympathize. We certainly can overdo this. I think that not only can we not fathom the complexity of the unconscious, but we don't need to do so. Like Tony with Dawn, we can understand from our knowledge of someone's past and help accordingly. Nonetheless, we should be aware that our behaviour is frequently influenced by unconscious mental forces. We may understand only some of this, but it can be helpful, as it is for me whenever I meet dogs.

Dog phobia

I hate dogs. Unconsciously. I try not to hate them consciously but I do struggle. And I know why. When I was a child our neighbours had a yappy, vicious dog. It bit me a couple of times on my legs. I wore welly boots when it was in the garden and on the loose. Then it bit me through my wellies! And then some years ago, when I was doing some door-to-door visitation near our church, a door opened to reveal what Sherlock Holmes might call a hound. A huge dog lunged out and bit a large chunk out of my coat as I legged it down the path.

So I know why I don't like dogs and why, when I meet them, I still get anxious and avoid them. I know that this is (largely) irrational, because most dogs are well trained and safe. Yet my fears still arise decades later. There are unconscious forces at work. It isn't really a phobia, as I can live life around dogs and get on with my life. But it illustrates how past events linger and affect us today. And how privileged I am that I never suffered anything worse.

Many others have suffered much worse. They have been scarred by wicked assaults. They have been damaged by abuse at the hands of parents or strangers. My dog phobia gives me a little insight into the difficulties many people have in living with the unconscious effects of such past horrible experiences. Like me, they may, to some extent, be conscious of these unconscious forces influencing their relationships today. This can help. But it doesn't make them go away and it is still hard work.

After her husband died Lorna became anxious. She had been with Jack as long as anyone could remember. Everyone knew how she relied on him. But they didn't know about her life before Jack. Her childhood had been one of poverty and neglect. She had had a mother who ignored her and an alcoholic father who beat her mother. And when she became a teenager he beat Lorna as well. Then in her late teens she met Jack. He became her rock, the only person she ever trusted and felt comfortable with. And so, with his death, her wariness of others emerged into the open as intense anxiety and emotional instability. She limps on with support from psychiatric services. But she doesn't have a Jack. And she has no church and no family either.

Forgiving and forgetting

Freudian theories want us to delve around and find the bad parenting and sinful influences that led to us forming bad habits. This approach encourages us to remember and think about such unhelpful matters. However, in doing this, these upsetting occasions become more real and more disturbing. This is why these approaches have proven to be failures.[12] This approach also conflicts with the Bible's teaching on forgiveness and reconciliation. In the parable of the unmerciful servant (Matthew 18:21–35) Jesus spelled out that Christians are to forgive without limit. The phrase 'not seven times, but seventy-seven times' (Matthew 18:22) means unlimited forgiveness.[13] The parable reinforces this point by adding that we should be so generously forgiving because we serve a God who has so abundantly forgiven us.

Thus, if we remember some incident in our childhood when someone mistreated us, we are called to forgive that person. Tony reminds Dawn about this when she feels resentful towards her parents. It isn't easy but it is important. We are not to seek to understand the mental mechanisms that have brought the memory back to us. We are certainly not to seek to uncover memories of bad events through psychotherapy. If this mistreatment has been repeated or horribly abusive, then forgiveness can be very difficult and repeated remembering will occur with associated mental pain.

Amy suffered at the hands of her alcoholic parents. She repeatedly harmed herself and abused alcohol and drugs. She struggled through her teens and twenties with a series of brief 'relationships' which further harmed her. She was befriended by generous Christians who helped her practically and emotionally and she came to faith. Her father had died when she was fifteen, but her mother lives on and Amy has worked hard at forgiveness. It is easier when Mum is elsewhere. But when Mum visits, the pain returns and she struggles with grim memories of physical and sexual abuse. The pain has eased over the years but will likely never disappear in this world.

The forgiveness approach does the opposite of Freudianism because it also includes 'forgetting' the incident, just as we are taught that God's forgiveness of us includes him casting our sins out of sight to be remembered no more (Psalm 103:11–12). Of course, God cannot actually forget, and we cannot wipe our memories clean. But our attitude should be that when memories of such bad events intrude into our consciousness, we banish them. We learn immediately to remind ourselves that we forgive that person's wickedness and we desire a constructive and mature relationship. Paul taught the Ephesians that the opposite of forgiveness is a bitter heart that leads to further retaliatory wickedness and divisions, whereas compassion and forgiveness heal and unite (Ephesians 4:31–32). Therefore, such forgiveness also aims at restoring relationships which may have been broken by such bad behaviour, just as God's forgiveness of us restores us to a relationship with him.

Carrying one another's burdens

Forgiveness can be tough. And it is about more than forgetting; it is about building and restoring relationships. This is tougher still, but is what we are taught in the New Testament. Peter teaches us that love covers over a multitude of sins (1 Peter 4:8). In our relationships we sin frequently. Sometimes, if you are like me, you may engage in that internal debate about whether it was a sin or not (by me or against me). Yet we know our deceitful hearts make this a hopeless exercise because we so easily trick ourselves. And so we forgive without limit and continue to love those who have sinned (or maybe not) against us. This love is practical. Like all loving in the Bible, it is primarily about actions. We continue to be kind towards and help those who have sinned (or maybe not) against us. Or, as Paul puts it to the Galatians, we carry one another's burdens as part of restoring relationships damaged by sin (Galatians 6:1–2).

The argument here is not that forgiveness and reconciliation in relationships is a therapy for mental illness. Such behaviour is right in itself and leads to better relationships in the present. And, God willing, it may lead to restored relationships with those who have hurt us in the past. How this biblical approach links with specialist treatments from psychiatric services is something we will look at in chapters 8 and 9. But now we need to consider (conscious) stress, the importance of which we observed earlier.

Key chapter points

- Much of our behaviour is unconsciously driven, and the Bible has a lot to say about this.
- The importance of the influence of the unconscious mind was made widely known by Sigmund Freud, but his models of the unconscious were flawed.
- Freudian approaches have been demonstrated to be unscientific and failures.
- The Bible gives us a surer guide to dealing with the influence of the unconscious mind.

5. STRESS AND CULTURE

Shell shock shocked everybody during the First World War. How could large numbers of strong, healthy men become crippled by afflictions with no physical cause? Tens of thousands were affected. No-one seemed exempt. Previously robust and well-balanced men suddenly developed blindness or paralysis, which self-evidently had no physical explanation. Men of officer class, as well as enlisted men, British, French, Austrian and German, all got shell shock. They developed the panoply of shell-shock symptoms – peculiar postures, blindness, deafness, paralysis in one arm, or both arms, or the legs. By the outbreak of the Second World War in 1939, 120,000 British soldiers had received awards for psychiatric disability related to shell shock, 40,000 were still drawing pensions and another 44,000 had received pensions for 'soldier's heart' (a related psychiatric condition).[1]

But what relevance is this to helping Christians today? To understand why many people develop mental illnesses we need to think further about the influence of the mind on the body. In the previous chapter we looked at the influence of the unconscious mind. Here we reflect on psychological stress and the ways in which societies and cultures shape the expression of illness symptoms. But rather than thinking this through theoretically, we will do so by reflecting on two historical phenomena which have important lessons for us today: shell shock and hysteria.

Shell shock

Shell shock was a broad term that covered a very large number of symptoms arising on the field of combat. While it was accepted that women could have such symptoms ('hysterical' symptoms, discussed further below), without physical disease pathology, the idea that men could have them too was astounding. Symptoms most commonly associated with shell shock were summarized by an Oxford Professor of Medicine writing home to a colleague in 1915: 'I wish you could be here in this orgy of neuroses and psychoses and gaits and paralyses. I cannot imagine what has got into the central nervous system of the men . . . hysterical dumbness, deafness, blindness, anaesthesia galore.'[2]

As the term implies, shell shock was initially thought to arise because of exposure to the damaging effects of exploding shells. The severity of the symptoms strongly suggested to soldiers and doctors alike that there must be a physical cause. However, sufferers usually had no signs of physical injury. And so it was proposed that maybe small fragments of shrapnel had damaged them. Or perhaps it was the concussive effects of exploding shells which had damaged the nervous system? Before long, though, it was conceded that there was no physical cause. Research found no evidence of the fragments or nervous damage. In fact, most men developing shell shock had not even been near exploding shells.

The reluctant disavowal of the physical damage interpretation opened up the way for a psychological explanation. This was, too often, only grudgingly accepted by both senior officers and doctors. There was a tendency among the military especially to argue that shell shock afflicted only the weak and feeble-minded. They wanted to believe that strong, sound men, especially those of the officer class, did not succumb to shell shock. Once again the evidence of their own eyes forced military officials and doctors to accept that this also was not correct. Everyone seemed to have his limit and could succumb to shell shock.

Fakes and frauds?

Why did these men develop shell shock? Were they frauds or sick? One view was that shell shock casualties were malingerers, who were shirking their duty to king and country, leaving their colleagues to face the heat of battle while they escaped to cosy safety. While it is clear that some men were consciously feigning symptoms, this was clearly not the case for the great majority.

Determining whether someone was faking illness as a malingerer or had genuine unconsciously driven symptoms was tricky. Charles Myers, a Jewish psychologist, stated, 'Between wilful cowardice, contributory negligence (i.e. want of effort against loss of self-control) and total irresponsibility for the shock, every stage and condition of shell shock may be found.'[3] Eventually most recognized that those enduring long periods of horrific levels of stress unconsciously developed their symptoms as a means of escaping the battlefield and gaining relief from it. After all, how else did you get out?[4] Escape could only come from death or injury on the battlefield, desertion and death by firing squad.

Many men shot themselves or exposed themselves by standing up to be shot, while others, unable to bear the strain, succumbed to shell shock. They became blind or lame and thus able to be relieved of their fighting duties. Blaming them for doing so was pointless and counterproductive since this simply put them under further stress. As Merskey observed, 'The miseries and hazards were substantial and the death rate enormous. At the same time popular feeling fiercely condemned men who would not fight, while the gallant wounded were praised and esteemed. It is hardly surprising that large numbers developed symptoms of illness without any organic foundation, so being honourably relieved of military service and perhaps even securing a pension.'[5]

Breaking points

No unified or sophisticated theories of shell shock were produced. And I doubt there can be. But there were several points on which there was agreement. The physical and psychological strain of trench warfare wore people down. Poor sleep night after night and exposure to artillery barrage day after day reduced soldiers to vulnerable levels of exhaustion. Seeing friends blown to pieces around them, being covered in soil from an exploding shell and left for dead on the battlefield could reduce many to tears. And the grim, un-remitting conditions in the trenches alone tested the mettle of the best of men. Eventually under this kind of strain perhaps anyone passed breaking point? Perhaps we all have breaking points? Maybe any of us exposed to such stress would succumb to some form of illness?

But it became clear that certain people were more vulnerable to shell shock than others. This vulnerability was individual, with some psychologically more susceptible ('mentally weaker') than others. But vulnerability also lay at a group level. Doctors observed that certain companies or divisions had much higher rates of shell shock than others. This was recognized to be due to the quality of leadership and morale, with badly led units being far more vulnerable to shell shock. Meanwhile, soldiers suffered the traumatic effects of warfare less acutely in well-led units that fostered good peer relationships. Similarly for us today, family and church are important aspects of life that can help to protect against stress-related symptoms and illness. Strong and supportive bonds help us because we are made to benefit from such relationships as God's image-bearers.

It isn't rocket science

The most effective treatments for shell shock involved rest reasonably near the frontline, sympathetic acknowledgment of the strain, and reassurance that the men did not have a serious, permanent illness but would swiftly recover. A period of rest relieved the physical and mental exhaustion. Doing so near the frontline reassured men that they would soon be able to resume combat alongside their comrades – an important assertion of confidence in them. The balance between a natural desire for self-preservation and duty to colleagues and country was tilted back to the latter. Acceptance that shell shock was an understandable response to the strain of war helped sufferers maintain their dignity and integrity. It was crucial to enabling them to have the morale needed to continue fighting. And encouraging them, by making it clear that they would get better and that they did not have irreversible brain damage, enabled them to get over their symptoms.

None of this required specialist expertise. Nor did it need a profound psychological understanding of why they got shell shock. This is just as well, as I suggested earlier, since no such understanding has ever emerged. But it did require a generous and compassionate attitude. An attitude that didn't blame and condemn, but desired to help and heal, the kind of Christian approach that we should be providing to the stressed and struggling, and especially to those who become disabled by mental illness. As they say, it isn't rocket science.

Cultural shift

In a culture where emotional expression was discouraged, men in their distress during the First World War developed disabling hysterical physical symptoms (the shell-shock phenomenon). Fifty years later, by the Vietnam War, the culture now permitted emotional symptoms. Stress did not need to produce paralysis and blindness any more. Stress could cause anxiety and sadness. Society allowed associated bodily features of distress too, such as pain, fatigue, sleeplessness and disturbed dreams. So post-traumatic stress disorder (PTSD) arose from the Vietnam War.

In his book *From Paralysis to Fatigue*[6] the medical historian Edward Shorter traces the shifts in the presentation of stress-related problems over the past couple of hundred years. Both wider cultural changes and shifts in medical conceptions of illness have affected how people respond to distress: 'In psychosomatic illness the body's response to stress or unhappiness is orchestrated by the unconscious. The unconscious mind, just like the conscious, is influenced by surrounding culture, which has models of what it considers to be legitimate and illegitimate symptoms.'[7] Cultural change clearly influenced how war stress was expressed by soldiers.

Nowadays stress more broadly produces a similar array of mental symptoms (such as anxiety, low mood, flashbacks and pessimism) and non-specific physical ones (fatigue, pains, appetite loss and poor sleep). These constitute the symptom patterns of the psychosomatic illnesses that we will consider in chapter 8.

Hysteria[8]

'How do you solve a problem like hysteria?' is not quite what the nuns sang in The Sound of Music. But it is a question that has been raised by successive generations of doctors. Today 'hysteria' might conjure up pop concerts with screaming teenagers or overexcited crowds. But, historically, hysteria referred to a broad category of illnesses having prominent mental and physical symptoms. That is, it referred to psycho-somatic illnesses.[9] It is a phenomenon that has puzzled physicians down the ages. A senior American neurologist even labelled it 'mysteria'.[10]

The wandering womb

The origins of hysteria are ancient, with descriptions in early Greek and Egyptian writings. The Greek physicians claimed that hysteria was caused by a 'wandering womb'. This, they thought, acted like a small animal roving around the body and damaging different bodily organs. It pushed upwards from the abdomen causing suffocation. It rose into the throat causing problems with swallowing. It pushed on the heart causing pain and so on. Later theories attributed symptoms to 'vapours' or 'nerves' (remember those fainting

Victorian women with their smelling salts, beloved of some novelists).

Much could be said about this, but the key point is that for many centuries hysteria was attributed to physical causes. The plethora of fluctuating bodily complaints was not dismissed as 'merely psychological'. Neither were hysterical symptoms regarded as fakery. There was never any question that the cause of hysteria lay in the body, from nerves or the womb.

Do people get hysteria today?

Whatever happened to hysteria?

Why did women seem to swoon a lot in the nineteenth century and they don't today? Why were smelling salts on hand when they are never found today? This is not merely biased selection. We find fascinating accounts in medical books and splendid examples in novels (and related films) from past centuries. So where do we find hysteria today?

Some people with 'classic hysteria' are still with us. Early in my psychiatric training I assessed a woman in a wheelchair. She claimed she had been unable to walk for a couple of years, having been paralysed following an accident at home. No-one had been able to clarify what this accident involved, although it did seem to be related to an argument about money. And this occurred in the context of family breakdown and thus mental stress. Physical examination revealed her nervous system was fine. Investigations, including scans of her brain and spine, confirmed the absence of pathology or damage.

Her paralysis had advantages. It had brought her family together to look after her. And her disability benefits gradually removed their debts. Had she then consciously chosen to fake her paralysis as a strategy to solve her family problems? Or was becoming paralysed an unconscious method for alleviating her distress in her home situation? It was clear that her paralysis had improved matters at home, since people tended now to focus on helping her rather than arguing.

Changing the clothing

The striking physical impairments caused by the myriad forms of classic hysteria – blindness, paralysis and so on – were a culturally acceptable way of expressing emotional distress. Men suffering in the trenches and women constrained by society's expectations 'broke down' into mental illness in this way. We noted above how the change in society in the twentieth century altered how soldiers responded to the stress of war. And just as shell shock morphed into PTSD as society changed, so hysteria has morphed into what we will call psychosomatic illness. I've chosen this term (which is also used by others in medicine) because it matches the biblical teaching on our psychosomatic wholeness.

Hysteria has always been understood to involve a combination of bodily symptoms and strong emotions. These emotions have typically been varying degrees of anxiety (including fear), depression and sometimes elation. The bodily symptoms have been vast and varied. They have involved every bodily organ – faints, a pounding heart, shortness of breath, blindness, paralysis, abdominal pains, difficulty in swallowing and tremors have been some of the most common. Hysteria was a psychosomatic type of illness: people with it had both physical and mental symptoms. And so today those with psychosomatic illnesses have a combination of physical and mental symptoms. But the type and pattern of these symptoms has changed, with mental symptoms becoming more prominent and physical ones less so. The outward form, the clothing, of stress-related illness has changed.

The power of the mind

Today it is widely assumed that all symptoms really come from the body. But it has only been in the past couple of hundred years that doctors have talked about symptoms as arising 'from the body', as if this could happen without the involvement also of the mind/soul. The influence of material-istic science has driven such a view, which conflicts with the biblical teaching on human beings as psychosomatic wholes.

We've seen that all illness involves body and soul. In the nineteenth and twentieth centuries there was widespread recognition that hysterical (psychosomatic) symptoms could arise from psychological mechanisms. Unfortunately, the growing influence of materialism meant that psychosomatic symptoms came to be thought of as 'merely' psychological. And for strongly biologically based neuroscience (my research work, incidentally) this implied they were not 'real'. Genuine symptoms were due to 'proper' organic (physical) illnesses, and psychosomatic illnesses were not real illnesses at all.

However, this dismissal of hysteria as 'not a proper illness', when it became conceived of as psychological in origin, has been difficult to sustain. Simon Wessely writes that the commonest view in society today 'is that these must be physical illnesses, not because of the evidence, which remains inconclusive, but because psychological illnesses are unreal, malingered or imaginary. This tendency of those committed to an exclusively organic view of such illnesses [is] to juxtapose psychiatric and imaginary.'[11]

This equation of psychiatric with imaginary or malingering is often found today. It contributes to the stigma of mental illness. The tension between the long-standing conviction that these people have real illnesses and the inability of modern science to explain them is a problem for materialists. But not once we accept a psychosomatic view of human beings in which mental mechanisms can powerfully affect bodily function.

Mad travellers

In his book *Mad Travelers*[12] Ian Hacking examines fugue states. These were hysterical conditions in which individuals disappeared on long journeys for weeks or months. They often journeyed to faraway places, claiming no memory of their earlier lives.[13] Hacking called fugue states 'the bodily expression of male powerlessness',[14] picking up the earlier phrase used to help explain hysteria in nineteenth-century women. He observed,

> The men have all sorts of problems, and they are curiously powerless in the face of their daily lives . . . their powerlessness which produces temporary mental breakdown, finds release in a mental illness which relieves them of responsibility, is cultured by medicine and is medicalised in the culture of the day, a culture that includes both tourism and vagrancy.[15]

Travelling like this when unable to cope with the mental stress at home and/or work was the only way out for these men. It was an escape mechanism for those lacking other means, other power, to get away. In the same way, historical hysteria can often be understood as a (usually) female escape mechanism from the rigid constraints of a difficult life. Similarly, and perhaps more obviously to us today, First World War soldiers became blind or paralysed because such dramatic physical symptoms were needed in order to escape the trenches. They provided a route to safety that was culturally acceptable in an era when to acknowledge anxiety, fear and exhaustion was not.

It is also clear that the symptoms of psychosomatic illnesses are strongly influenced by personal experience, as well as the surrounding culture. Good relationships at work (as with well-led units of soldiers) protect us against such illnesses; by extension, this is so too for positive relationships in church and elsewhere. And 'simple' approaches to treatment (rest, peer support, encouragement) can be very effective, as they were for shell shock. Thus, again, we see the importance of both of our two image-related functions: rule and relationships. These can furnish protection from mental illnesses (reducing vulnerability) and provide effective approaches to caring for people with such illnesses.

New stress, new clothing

As we know by now, culture shapes the expression of mental and physical symptoms. The modern shift towards permitting emotional expression has changed how psychosomatic illnesses manifest themselves. We saw this in the changes in how soldiers reacted to stress. Social constraints and class structures led them to 'escape into illness' (to simplify). Today men and women, at least in the West, have much greater freedom to develop and express their God-given abilities. Escaping stress does not require us to develop fugues or other forms of classic hysteria.

But stress remains. Other cultural pressures have replaced those of the past. People try to juggle careers and family life, feeling the pressure to hold down jobs to pay the rent or mortgage, while ferrying kids to school. Others are sandwiched between the burden of caring for elderly parents, perhaps far away, and supporting adult children trying to make their way in an unstable and rapidly changing job market. And then there are the more dubious cultural pressures to conform to: the obsession with wealth, appearance and material goods. Such stresses can produce psychosomatic illnesses today.

But the clothing of these has changed. Today emotion is allowed to be prominent. We can cry. We can be sad. We can express our fears. The psychosomatic illnesses of today are dominated by such mental symptoms. They are called anxiety disorders, somatic (body) symptom disorders and stressor-related disorders. But these categories are unstable. People move from one to the other and between the many diagnoses within them. And so they are widely criticized as not meaningful terms. Hence, for the purposes of this book, I refer to them all as psychosomatic illnesses. They share the same kinds of cause and the same fluctuating array of mental and physical symptoms.

A biased book

I have a confession to make. This book is biased. But I have biased it against my own interests. My research largely involves brain tissue, brain imaging and studies of molecules and biology. And yet, I have not commented on the biology of mental illnesses. This is not because I am uninterested in this. Or because it is unimportant. And certainly not because we lack evidence. Rather, to discuss this properly requires dealing with many specialist areas of neuroscience, which takes us way beyond the scope of this book.

Summarizing and simplifying, a wealth of evidence (from genetic, brain imaging and many other studies) demonstrates that the severe mental illnesses (chapter 9) contain a large biological component, while the psychosomatic illnesses have a smaller biological contribution. So, for example, particular genes and early physical ill health make some people highly vulnerable to developing schizophrenia. And stress plays a minor role in such people becoming ill, or perhaps none at all (as with Alison whom we'll meet below). 'Anxiety disorders' (within the psychosomatic class) have a large proportion of stress-related causation. But they also have some important neurobiological vulnerability.

Alison had been stable for years on antipsychotics for her schizophrenia. She had grown older and her care was passed to me, but I rarely saw her. I didn't need to because she was so well. At times I wondered about stopping her treatment (but whenever I have done this for such people, they have got ill again and so I didn't). She was regularly seen by a community nurse (who would discuss her with me), and I would occasionally visit. Then one day I got an urgent phone call. She had locked herself in her house and was terrified about the ghosts that were interfering with her mind and trying to make her attack her neighbours. We admitted her. She was physically well and there were no recent changes in her life. We couldn't identify any stressors to explain why she had now become ill again. Presumably, her mental illness worsened in her brain as diseases do. I'm glad to say she recovered well with changes to her treatment.

Stress-vulnerability model of mental illness

Finally, we come to consider a common, and necessarily simplified, approach to thinking about the causation of mental illness: the stress-vulnerability model. This proposes that people have a varying degree of vulnerability to illness, which makes them prone to developing mental illnesses under differing amounts of physical and psychological stress. In the stress-vulnerability model an episode of illness is triggered by some stressor that acts upon the person. This pushes individuals beyond their limits of coping so they become dysfunctional and distressed. Or, in the language of our definition of mental illness, it produces 'clinically significant impairment in everyday functioning'.

Within the overall stress-vulnerability model it is the combination of physical/biological and psychological predisposition that renders people more or less vulnerable to illness episodes. That is, we are vulnerable as psychosomatic whole persons. The impact of a complex array of psychological factors upon us can induce an episode of illness. Factors such as relationship stress at work or illness in a loved one at home may precipitate mental illness. Similarly, episodes of illness may be induced by physical factors. These may be brain changes due to underlying biological disease or the bodily impact of non-brain physical illnesses. The type and pattern of illness are determined by our specific stress-vulnerability; we are individually prone to different types of illness.

Jude had struggled in coping with recent changes in his workplace and went to his GP with stress. His GP arranged for some counselling at the practice, but before this got started Jude had an accident and fractured his leg. He was admitted to hospital for an operation, which was complicated by a bad post-operative infection. But everything was further complicated by Jude becoming severely depressed and needing to be transferred to inpatient psychiatric care. He eventually made a full recovery on a combination of antidepressants and with nursing support and CBT (cognitive-behavioural therapy) at home. Was this severe depression due to the physical stress of his fracture and infection? Or the psychological stress of becoming seriously ill on top of the chronic workplace difficulties? We know that both interact and both were likely to have been significant for Jude's depression.

An important benefit of understanding the causes of an illness is that it can help us to direct our treatment more appropriately. In Jude's case, as is very common, both physical (antidepressant) and psychological (CBT and support) treatments were helpful because both physical and psychological factors contributed to his illness. Oversimplifying, illnesses that are more biological require treatments that are more heavily biological. Thus for schizophrenia, antipsychotic medication is the mainstay of treatment, especially in acute episodes. But specific psychological treatments, especially CBT, can be helpful alongside a structured and supportive social network. Here support from people in church can also be particularly important (see chapters 8 and 9).

Vulnerability

It is more usual when thinking about human development and the acquisition of robust or fragile personalities to focus on major traumatic events: personal injury, rape, physical abuse and so on. Such horrific experiences do cause serious damage, especially during childhood, rendering people vulnerable to mental illnesses. And it is also sadly true that most of these horrific childhood experiences occur in the larger context of a grim childhood saturated with criticism and many lesser hardships.

A young girl who is sexually abused by her mother's boyfriend has typically endured such abuse on many occasions, not as a one-off experience. Even worse, she is likely to have endured this as part of a childhood characterized by bullying, neglect, daily family arguments and violence. The extent of psychological damage in such circumstances can be severe, leaving her with no assurance about herself, no confidence in relationships, especially with men, and a desperate need for companionship.

Here is not the place to be specific or to repeat examples of gruesome experiences, for the point is a simple one: experiences, especially in childhood, shape our personalities. Bad experiences misshape us. This makes us liable to mental illnesses later in life. But it is important not to forget the impact of the drip-drip-drip of a grim home environment. A boy who is repeatedly criticized at home, apparently randomly, and largely ignored by his parents, grows to be uncertain and needing emotional assurance elsewhere. Thus at school he attempts to engage with the premier league gossip. But because his feckless father hasn't even talked to him about the football that he spends so much time watching, he is exposed as ignorant. And he is ridiculed and runs away in tears, a little more damaged. The psychological fragility he has acquired at home is worsened. It is by a multitude of such inter-personal interactions and life experiences that each of us is shaped; that is, we acquire our own level of emotional stability and responsiveness or, as with this boy, our own degree of personal vulnerability.

Stressful experiences

So our upbringing and experiences build on our biological make-up and make us more, or less, vulnerable to mental illnesses by leaving us as more, or less, damaged persons. Again, we tend to think of major stressors precipitating illness episodes, events that have a large emotional impact, such as the loss of a loved one, redundancy or a physical assault. Such experiences do place great strain on us and can tip many into an illness, even those with a previously stronger constitution.

But the drip, drip, drip of chronic difficulties can also wear us down so that eventually we can no longer cope and we develop a psychosomatic illness. This seems to have been the case for many with shell shock who succumbed without ever being in the trenches. In such circumstances it can be difficult to identify the trigger because several factors combine together until a tipping point is reached.

The same kind of personal events and experiences contributes to both vulnerability and stress. However, it is generally useful to distinguish between long-standing vulnerability and more recent stressors precipitating illness episodes. Vulnerability points us to our knowledge of the person in the long term and the main life events that have shaped them. Stress clearly relates to current or recent events. Usually such stressors are easier to identify and deal with than personal vulnerability from the lingering effects of the past. This is not to say it is easy, though. Ultimately, in this world we won't be able to undo much of the damage inflicted and we look to our future and deliverance from all this through Christ.

Mental illness or distress?

We have just sketched out an approach to understanding and helping people. It should be obvious by now that stressors act upon us to induce understandable distress. For people with milder levels of distress, then support and constructive practical input from a church (and family and friends) may be sufficient to restore them. (We will discuss this at length in the stepped-care approach in chapter 8.)

But when the stressful load is large enough, it overwhelms us so we cease to cope normally, and our distress becomes clinically significant. It becomes illness, and those with illness need input from primary care or psychiatric services. But the role of the church family and others still remains crucial. When someone becomes mentally ill and specialist input is needed from health services, the church should not withdraw. The input of Christians should be an important component of the care of the mentally ill.

The stress-vulnerability model is applicable whether the person is distressed or ill. Milder and borderline cases can undoubtedly benefit greatly from personal support and practical help in our churches. Ministers and other mature Christians are very well equipped to handle these kinds of problems. The church family should be able to provide practical and personal support.

When someone crosses the threshold into illness, Christians in churches can usefully work closely with health professionals. As a church, we don't simply hand people over to primary care or psychiatric services. We should work with them. With such Christians we have established relationships and a long-term understanding of the whole person. This provides us as church leaders with an excellent starting position. It enables the church family to contribute throughout, even when medical services become involved.

Key chapter points

- Stress and traumatic experience exert a powerful influence on our being.
- This can cause mental illnesses in people of all types through conscious and unconscious mechanisms.
- The symptoms and pattern of such illnesses are shaped by our personalities and by our culture.
- Biological mechanisms are also very important in generating mental illnesses.

6. PERSONAL RESPONSIBILITY AND MENTAL ILLNESS

Mr A was an eighty-one-year-old in a nursing home whom I was asked to assess because he had 'repeatedly sexually assaulted a female resident'. Clinical assessment revealed he had a dementia due to Alzheimer's disease, and he believed the female victim to be his wife who in fact had died four years earlier.

Mr B suffered a stroke and, as a result, had a vascular dementia. The police were called some months later because he had inflicted several deep lacerations on his wife with a knife. I was asked to assess whether he knew what he was doing and was consequently to blame for this knife crime.

Mrs C was a forty-four-year-old whom I assessed after she had attacked some teenage children – some neighbours' kids had strayed into her garden. Fortunately no serious injuries occurred. It became clear she had paranoid schizophrenia, having been increasingly plagued for weeks by fears that her neighbours were spying on her and conspiring to kill her.

Mrs D was a fifty-one-year-old on antidepressants and receiving CBT for her depressive illness. I was summoned urgently by her daughter after she had whacked her husband and thrown hot tea over him. Her husband had called the police who had subsequently arrested him! She was in tears when I arrived, as was her daughter.

These four each suffered from a mental illness. Each had committed potential crimes in the view of the state. And sins against God. Or had they? Were they guilty of crimes or sins? Before answering such questions, we need to review the scriptural teaching on sin and responsibility.

Sickness and sin

We have seen that mental illness is a behavioural syndrome resulting from a response to some objective cause (external or internal). This cause may be physical or psychological. And the clinical symptoms produce significant impairment in everyday functioning. But what is sin? Sin is evil. But not any kind of evil. Sin is a moral evil. Sickness may be regarded as an 'evil' in the broad sense of the badness that results from the fall, but it is not a moral evil. Theologian Louis Berkhof observes, 'It is possible to speak not only of sin but also of sickness as an evil, but then the word "evil" is used in two totally different senses.'[1]

Sickness and sin are separate concepts which are defined in different ways. Psychiatrist Andrew Sims observes,

In trying to decide what is and what is not mental illness it is useful to consider different dimensions, for example, contrasting the mentally ill and the mentally healthy. An entirely separate and independent dimension is good/bad or right/wrong. That these variables are independent of each other is obvious but it does need stating.[2]

Sin operates in the moral sphere of behaviour. The essence of sin is that it is behaviour that is contrary to the law and character of God (e.g. Romans 1:18–32; 1 John 3:4). Wayne Grudem defines sin as 'any failure to conform to the moral law of God in act, attitude or nature'.[3] It is not transgression of our conventions or social practice. It is not behaviour that I don't like in someone else. It is not bizarre actions or emotionally distressed behaviour that upsets me. People with mental illness do all these things. But they aren't sins unless God's law is broken.

Illness and sin are in different conceptual categories. My moral behaviour is evaluated against God's standards of right and wrong. When I transgress these in thought, word or deed, then I sin against God. Such behaviour is my behaviour and I am responsible for it. This applies whether my behaviour is conscious or unconscious. The great majority of my sin is unconscious.

But illness results from events that happen to me and for which I am not responsible. When ill I may behave righteously in seeking God's face in prayer and desiring to be made more like Christ through the trial of my illness. Or due to fatigue and increased susceptibility to irritable behaviour I may speak rudely to my wife and thus sin.

As Christians we need to remind ourselves that all sorts of words and deeds are legitimate and can be said and done to the praise and honour of God (1 Corinthians 10:31; Colossians 3:17). There seems to be a perennial tendency to create a narrow field of right Christian conduct. Any kind of distressed behaviour easily becomes classified as sinful because it has crossed these unbiblically tiny boundaries. Broken souls, people disabled by mental illness, are not able to function efficiently. But their struggle to cope should not lead to the conclusion that they have sinned or are sinning. Like the psalmists in their anguish, they may be trusting in Christ and aiming to walk with him during their emotional pain.

Individual responsibility in the Bible

From Genesis to Revelation the Scriptures present a clear and consistent position on personal responsibility: each of us is individually accountable to God for all our behaviour. Good or bad. During the exile, the Israelites complained that they were being unjustly punished by God. They moaned, 'The parents eat sour grapes, and the children's teeth are set on edge' (Ezekiel 18:2). The Lord responded with the clearest statement of individual responsibility in the Bible (Ezekiel 18:1–18).[4]

Here Ezekiel sketches out three generations: a righteous father who abhors the rampant idolatry, sexual immorality, abuse of power and maltreatment of the poor so characteristic of his peers; his son, who indulges in idolatry, adultery, murder and robbery; and his grandson, who mirrors his grandfather's behaviour in faithfully serving the Lord by caring for the poor, shunning idols and being faithful in marriage. And the point is repeated. Each will die for his or her own sin: 'The one who sins is the one who will die' (Ezekiel 18:20). This is the consistent biblical position. Everyone is punished for his or her own bad behaviour and not for anyone else's wickedness.

Parents and genes are not excuses

But there is more here, isn't there? For we see that people's genes, upbringing and social context provide no excuse for their wickedness. These three generations shared the same genes (or at least a lot of them, 50% down each generation).

They lived in the same wicked environment in the Babylonian Empire. And yet their lifestyle changed from generation to generation.

The wicked son ignored his father's teaching on serving the Lord. He disobeyed and turned away from God to run after idols and break other commandments. In spite of this dreadful example and lack of training by his father in the ways of the Lord, the grandson lived uprightly, keeping the laws of the Lord and obeying him from his heart.[5]

So children who are wicked are punished even though they may be following the example of their parents; bad parenting provides no excuse for anyone to sin. In fact, the Scriptures warn us against not punishing sin because to do so encourages others to follow in wickedness. Tremper Longman comments on Ecclesiastes 8:11 that the preacher 'asserts that when there is no apparent punishment for evil, then it will flourish. If people do not observe negative consequences for bad actions, they will be encouraged to do more evil.'[6] This observation of the preacher has often been repeated down the ages when wrong-doing has been allowed to go unpunished by those in authority.

Illness and responsibility

So we see that the Bible teaches a robust position on individual responsibility. We are not allowed to shift the blame to our genes, or our parents, or our horrible experiences, or our bad social environment, or the bad influence of peers. Or to our illness. We do not choose to be ill. But we make choices when ill for which we are responsible. Nowhere in Scripture does such sickness excuse us from our transgressions. When King Ahaziah was ill, following a fall from a window, his wicked, idolatrous behaviour was condemned by the Lord through his prophet Elijah (2 Kings 1). His sickness was severe enough to confine him to bed and kill him. But this terminal illness did not absolve him from his sin.

When I have the flu, I feel rotten and become more irritable. But if I lose my temper and shout at my children, then I have sinned. I am not excused because I was sick and thus more prone to sin. Rather, when sick, I need to be especially careful and to pray more fervently for self-control so I don't dishonour the Lord by such outbursts. We all know that when in pain or discomfort, when fatigued or febrile, we are more vulnerable to temptations to sin. So illness, even severe illness like that of Ahaziah, does not excuse us for our sins when ill. But what about the mentally ill?

Mental capacity

Throughout history it has been recognized that to be guilty we need to be able to recognize the difference between right and wrong. We need to understand what we are doing and to be aware that such an action is morally wrong. Norman Geisler summarizes this as 'morality follows upon rationality'.[7]

In English common law the Latin phrase *mens rea* (guilty mind) has long been used in relation to crimes to refer to the necessity of the person not only having committed the criminal act (*actus reus*), but also having had the mental capacity to know that this behaviour was wrong. To be convicted of a crime requires both the act and the mental intention to do wrong. So if someone lacks the mental ability to understand his or her action and to recognize it as a crime, then that person cannot be found guilty.

In the Old Testament, Isaiah speaks in 7:15–16 of a boy reaching the stage of being able to 'refuse the evil and choose the good' (ESV). He is old enough to know the difference between morally good and bad behaviour and is responsible for deciding accordingly.[8] A complementary aspect to this ability to discern right from wrong is the necessity of having the right information to make a decision. We see this in Jonah 4:11. Here the Lord rebukes Jonah for his callous attitude to Nineveh. He tells him he should have pity, as the Lord has, for the 120,000 people in Nineveh who 'cannot tell their right hand from their left'. The point here is not that Nineveh contained a vast number of infants, but that the Ninevites lacked the knowledge that God was going to destroy them. They were ignorant of his proposed destruction of their city. He had sent a reluctant Jonah to warn them and so they had repented. They were a people who had the mental capacity to know right from wrong, but they lacked the necessary information to act. The Lord had pity by giving them this warning and so brought them to repentance.[9] These are the two key elements: to be guilty of sin we must be given the knowledge that an act is sinful, and we must have the relevant mental capacity to understand that available knowledge.[10]

Not guilty by reason of insanity

Let us move on to mental illness and legal accountability. Historically, the insanity defence was developed in England following the acquittal of Daniel McNaughton of the murder of Edward Drummond, secretary to Prime Minister Robert Peel, in 1843. McNaughton was a Scottish craftsman who suffered from delusions, and the McNaughton (or M'Naghten) rules were formulated by judges after this trial and have since been used, in various legal jurisdictions, to enable someone to be declared 'not guilty by reason of insanity'.

The key elements of the insanity defence are that defendants are assumed to be sane unless the contrary is proven. And they must be shown to have a 'disease of the mind' which resulted either in them not knowing what they were doing, or if they did, not knowing that it was wrong (mental capacity and relevant information again). Thus the mere presence of a mental illness is not a sufficient defence. It needs to be severe enough to damage the reasoning process so that the sufferer does not understand the meaning of his or her behaviour. And the person also needs to have the understanding that such a behaviour constitutes a crime. The interpretation of these McNaughton rules by courts of law has been complex, and sometimes controversial, and is well beyond our scope here.[11] But in general terms their development formalized the long-standing recognition that people could be found not guilty because of the effect of mental illness.

More recently, and more broadly, the language of 'mental capacity' (or in some places 'mental competence') has been used for determining the impact of mental illness on decision-making ability. There is consistency across countries in recognizing that four elements are required for individuals to be deemed to have the mental capacity to make decisions: they must be able to understand the relevant information; retain/remember this information; weigh it up to arrive at a decision; and communicate the decision to others.

Again, in mental capacity legislation the capacity to make decisions and the responsibility for such decisions is assumed to be present unless proven otherwise. And the relevant knowledge to form a decision and take an action must be, or have been, available to the person. So let us take an everyday example for me.

Making stupid decisions

When I prescribe a drug, I explain the benefits expected from taking the treatment and the likely adverse effects. The mentally competent adult understands what I've said, might ask some questions, thinks it over and decides . . . not to take the drug. If I have any doubts about the mental capacity of my patient, I should formally assess this using the four criteria. But otherwise I accept his or her decision, even when I don't like it. Or think it stupid.

The good news is that you are allowed to make stupid decisions. As we know, people with full mental capacity do silly things. And that is OK. It is your decision. It is sometimes joked that doctors will only deem someone mentally competent if they agree with a patient's decision. But this is not so (or at least should not be so). I raise this to highlight that the decision-making process is distinguished from the decision itself. Those with mental capacity are free to make what I, or any doctor, might regard as a foolish decision. As long as they demonstrate they can understand, retain, weigh up and communicate their decision, they can decide to go bungee jumping or paragliding or anything else I regard as stupid.

Although I am recognized as an expert in making such decisions, I confess I have prescribed for a mentally incompetent individual without following this principle. I once wrote a prescription for an antipsychotic for a patient, only to be urgently called back a few days later. My patient was now much more distressed by her delusions. But I discovered that her dog had received the antipsychotic (without any capacity assessment!) and she had taken the dog's steroids. She settled quickly on the correct medication. The dog was not harmed in the production of this anecdote.

Getting married is easy

Another important principle about decision-making is proportionality. Some decisions are more complex than others and so require a higher degree of mental capacity. In other words, capacity is not black and white but grey. You may be capable of making some decisions but not more complex ones.

And the issue here is complexity, not importance. Getting married is an important decision. But an easy one (at least regarding mental capacity!). It is simple because what marriage involves is generally well known without the need for lots of extra information and special expertise. Thus, some people with learning disability can marry, even though they may lack the capacity for more complex decisions such as managing their finances.

To return to medicine. To decide whether or not to take the antidepressant I prescribe is a straightforward decision. But the same person who has the capacity for such a decision may simultaneously not be able to decide whether or not to undergo a complex surgical procedure or to receive psychotherapy, because these require a higher level of mental capacity. Hence, decisions about capacity must be made on a case-by-case basis.

The same capacity principles apply to sinful (or criminal) behaviour. People are assumed to be capable of making moral decisions unless there is good reason to doubt this. There are two categories of people who may lack such mental capacity: children and the mentally ill. For children, different societies have declared different ages at which they become criminally responsible, and different ages at which they are deemed capable of making other decisions.

In England and Wales, for example, the age of criminal responsibility is ten, while you can decide to marry at sixteen (with parental consent), drive a car at seventeen and vote at eighteen. This has often been ridiculed as absurdly inconsistent. In fact, it broadly reflects the principle of proportionality. Voting is the most complex of these decisions, requiring the highest level of capacity; driving a car requires more decision-making ability than getting married (a relatively simple decision, as we've seen). Knowing right from wrong behaviour, and thus bearing criminal responsibility, is the easiest of all.

Sinning is easy

The last point is key here. Moral decisions are the easiest. And so not to be responsible you have to be very impaired mentally. The Scriptures teach us we have God's moral law written on our hearts (Romans 2:14–16). We all know certain behaviours (stealing, lying, assault, adultery and so on) are sinful. It doesn't matter whether or not any particular country declares them also to be a crime. The knowledge of what is morally right and wrong is available to everyone. So, like marriage, sinning is an easy decision. Even easier. From birth we have the information on right and wrong because God has written it inside us. It is simple to grasp, and the knowledge of right and wrong is there all our lives.

We've seen that societies generally have regarded some people with mental illness as not mentally competent and so not responsible for their criminal and, by extension, sinful actions. The limited biblical data seems to support this position. But to lose capacity for moral decisions requires a large loss of capacity because these are simple decisions. In other words, you have to be severely mentally ill to have lost such moral capacity. How ill? Well, there is no easy answer. It is a case-by-case matter. Let me stick my neck out and attempt to be a bit more specific.

Sticking my neck out

What kinds of mental illness might render someone incapable of making a competent moral decision? In my opinion the answer falls into four broad categories of mental illness: mental handicap, psychosis, delirium and dementia. So I think that people suffering from other kinds of mental illness are mentally competent and are (perhaps with very rare exceptions) responsible for their sins (and crimes).

Let's return to the examples with which I opened this chapter. Mr A was not guilty of sexual sin. He had a severe dementia and could not comprehend that his actions might be wrong. But also, because of his dementia, he had a relevant delusion. He believed the woman he was molesting was his wife. (We call this 'delusional misidentification', a common feature of dementia.) Thus, he thought the female resident in his nursing home was his wife and so he treated her as if she were his wife.

On the other hand, Mr B was guilty of sin. He was breaking the sixth commandment by assaulting his wife. Although he had a dementia, this was mild and he understood his actions and knew them to be wrong. In fact, he was arrested by the police and charged when I declared he had capacity. The charges were later dropped, but the experience of being held in custody chastised him. He never assaulted his wife again.

People with dementia and mental handicap who lack such capacity will not recover it. This is the key difference with delirium and psychosis – people with these can recover. Delirium is a syndrome of short-term global brain impairment which, like dementia, usually occurs in older people. It differs from dementia by its brief duration and rapid onset. It has a wide range of causes, such as severe bodily illnesses and intoxication by drugs, and is especially common in hospital. When you visit someone in hospital, you will often find that person has become very confused. This is 'delirium'. The patient is temporarily incapacitated and sometimes, as with severe dementia and mental handicap, will have lost capacity for moral decision-making.

Psychosis is an umbrella term rather than a diagnosis. Psychosis occurs in severe mental illnesses (schizophrenia, depression or bipolar disorder) and causes people to be detached from reality and thus unable to engage in rational thinking. It also occurs in mental handicap and dementia. You will have noticed that Mr A lacked capacity due to both psychosis and mental impairment because of his dementia. Mrs C was not guilty of crime or sin in my opinion. Her reasoning was deranged by her schizophrenia, and she was deluded and convinced that she was being attacked. She had acted in self-defence as she understood it.

It is important to emphasize that such incapacity/ incompetence is not a necessary consequence of having any of these conditions. Most people, most of the time, will be capable even when they have these illnesses. Of course, each capacity decision needs to be made on a case-by-case basis.

Excusing sin

One reason why Christians sometimes find it difficult to accept mental illnesses, such as depression, is that the diagnosis has been used to excuse sin. But people are sinning all the time! People sin in sickness and in health. A man who has not returned to work may be shirking, using his depression after his redundancy as an excuse for sinful idleness (1 Thessalonians 5:14). He may shout rudely at his wife and blame this on 'the illness'. But he has capacity, he knows what he is doing and is guilty.

However, we should also acknowledge that troubled souls suffering from mental illnesses are vulnerable to sinful temptations. They need compassion and help. Sin is not excused, but neither is coldness and lack of sympathy. There is no contradiction in blaming them for their sin while also expressing compassion and offering help. Rather the opposite – we should be both firm on responsibility for sin, and kind to them, supporting them and counselling them for their mental illness.

Mrs D was guilty of sinful behaviour. Although depressed, she understood what she was doing and knew it was wrong. She told me she was sorry. I said that I understood it was difficult because she wasn't well and I encouraged her to see her community nurse more often. I increased the anti-depressants because she was not dealing well with her depression. And I asked her to contact the police and explain that she had acted badly and it was her fault. Her husband came home and she apologized to him (although it was not a happy ending as she has repeated similar behaviour since).

A good catch-22

The principal reason for discussing this topic has been to help church leaders and lay members involved in pastoral care. I want you to be more confident that we can, and should, hold people accountable for their sin even when they are ill. This is right, and should be done with care and compassion. But our consideration of personal responsibility has led us to a catch-22 situation.

I've encountered many people using their mental illness as an excuse for sin. But they all had capacity and were guilty. However, I've never met anyone who lacks capacity using this excuse. And they wouldn't, would they? Those who are so mentally impaired that they lack moral capacity will always also lack the mental capacity to try to take advantage of their illness in this way. Any who claim to lack capacity have it and so can't be excused their sin. Those who don't have capacity don't make such excuses. Such catch-22 situations are usually bad, with people trapped by bureaucratic power-plays. But this is a good one.

The sin-excuser's paradox

We can see that capacity and responsibility are important morally and pastorally. But does it make any difference medically? Yes. A huge difference. You are ill with depression. And Professor Thomas comes along and declares you lack capacity for your behaviour. But this means you must also lack capacity for all aspects of your care and treatment, since these are easier decisions. So now you no longer get to decide which treatments you will receive. Or who looks after you. Or where you are treated. Instead, big (actually small), bad Professor Thomas gets to make them all for you. Just as he does with people with severe dementia or schizophrenia.

This is the sin-excuser's paradox. If you are severely impaired enough to be excused for moral behaviour, then you are also incapable of making any of the everyday decisions we take for granted. Anyone genuinely severely impaired enough to lack moral capacity will also be too impaired to make simpler decisions about their care and treatment. Of course, people pretend it is the other way around. They can be excused for bad behaviour but are still free to make all the decisions they want about everything else. But not so. To be consistent, the sin-excuser must give up all decision-making.

But positively, this means that the great majority of people with mental illnesses are capable of participating in their care and treatment. They have enough mental capacity to join in deciding about all the important aspects of their treatment.

And so we can deal with them as responsible human beings who enjoy that dignity and respect that we all should receive as image-bearers.

Key chapter points

- The Bible clearly teaches that human beings are personally responsible for our actions and accountable ultimately to God.
- Different countries share common approaches to determining the level of responsibility of people with mental illnesses for their behaviour.
- These recognize that sometimes the impact of mental illness leaves someone lacking the mental capacity to make decisions.
- This includes moral decisions and fits with the Bible's teaching that in some circumstances people are not morally responsible for their individual acts.
- But most people with mental illness are responsible for their behaviour most of the time.

7. DRUGS, ECT AND PSYCHOTHERAPY

Malcolm was raging and fighting invisible men when I entered the ward. Invisible to me. But not to him. He had dementia with distressing visual hallucinations. He was injuring staff and patients in his rage, believing he was defending himself and others against assaults. He didn't know where he was or what we were doing when trying to help him. I had brought him to hospital for treatment under the Mental Health Act after he had caused havoc in his neighbourhood attacking the hallucinations he believed were persecuting him. But he took the donepezil (an anti-dementia drug) and improved a little. And as he took higher doses, he got better and better. I increased the dose again just before I went away with my family on holiday.

When I returned to the ward a couple of weeks later, Malcolm greeted me, asking, 'Excuse me, are you a doctor? Could you tell me why I am here?' I was stunned. His memory was normal. He had no hallucinations. He was completely well again.

Effective or ineffective treatments?

All the major categories of psychiatric treatment (the drugs, ECT and psychotherapies of this chapter title) have been criticized as ineffective or immoral or dangerous. So we will now reflect a little on how we learn whether treatments are beneficial and safe (and moral).

The treatment paradox

Malcolm illustrates well a problem we have with obtaining research to provide evidence that treatments work. How could you have entered Malcolm into a research study? He was far too aggressive and distressed to participate in a drug trial. The paradox of medical research, especially in psychiatry, is that the most severely ill people like Malcolm can't help us find evidence about the effectiveness of treatments. We can only study people who are less ill.

There is a lot of evidence from research trials that the more severely ill you are, the better you do with treatment. This is true for drugs and psychotherapies. But it isn't surprising, is it? The more ill you are, the more you can improve. However, since only people with mild and moderate illnesses enter studies, this means we see only small benefits from treatment. It gives the impression that the treatments are much less beneficial than they are.

Snake oil

Over the centuries all sorts of pills and potions have been sold as 'treatments' by quacks. Today it is often claimed that standard psychiatric treatments don't work. In effect we psychiatrists are said to be twenty-first-century peddlers of snake oil. How do we work out if a treatment really is effective? The late journalist John Diamond was forced to face the snake-oil question when he contracted throat cancer. Learning of his illness, many people contacted him offering a bewildering variety of cures. He ended up writing a book *Snake Oil*, a moving and highly readable summary of how we get medical evidence that treatments work, or don't.

The best evidence that treatments in medicine work comes from randomized, double-blind clinical trials using placebos.[1] Randomizing means I can't choose who gets what, otherwise I would give my favourite drug to people I knew from experience would do well anyway. Blinding means the patient doesn't know who received which treatment. Double-blinding means I don't know either: the placebo and drug tablets look the same.[2] A placebo is a 'sugar pill' and so should do nothing. But it isn't so simple.

The power of placebo

Placebos are interesting. I enjoy talking about them and asking, 'Why have placebos got better and better over the past thirty years?' Answer: changes in how drug trials are conducted. But you might now ask, 'If placebos are getting more powerful, then surely they aren't inert after all? Don't they do something?' Correct. People receiving placebos do a lot better than those who receive nothing at all.[3]

Research on the 'placebo effect' shows that much of their benefit comes from contact with research nurses. In drug trials research nurses regularly visit everyone to check how they are doing. They are very nice people. They bring kindness and understanding and words of sympathy to everyone in the study. Recent evidence shows that the more visits you have from research nurses, the better you get.[4] Much of the power of placebo lies in this non-specific support given by such nurses. They really do help people get better. Without trying.

It is important we note that these nurses are not doing any specific therapy at all. Sometimes they are told not to try to be helpful! They are just to check up on progress. But merely having kind, warm and sympathetic people visiting regularly really helps. And this is why people from churches can make a difference. You will bring the same kind of warmth and sympathy. This really will help those with mental illnesses improve. And that is without even trying to bring the wise counsel and advice we discuss below. And, of course, prayer.

Psychiatric drugs

There are only a few classes of psychiatric drugs in common use: antidepressants, antipsychotics, mood stabilizers, anxiolytics (anti-anxiety drugs), hypnotics (sleeping tablets), antidementia drugs and psychostimulants. The first five groups are used in people of all ages, while the last two are used in specific conditions that are strongly age-related: dementia (usually in older people) and attention-deficit/hyperactivity disorder[5] (ADHD, normally used in children). Within each class there are sometimes a large number of individual drugs.

Contrary to oft-repeated claims, there is robust evidence from randomized clinical trials that these drugs are effective and safe. Some of this evidence will be considered later. The real questions are how much they help and how much they harm (since all treatments have side effects). And thus how ill does someone need to be to justify using them. We will consider some of these questions in chapter 9 when we look at individual severe mental illnesses. But here we now consider not the scientific questions about psychiatric medication, but the ethical question: are such drugs morally acceptable for Christians?

Is it immoral to use 'mind-altering drugs'?

I hope you think this is an odd question. But aspersions have been cast on psychiatric drugs. We are told they are bad because they are 'mind-altering'. Or they are merely 'general sedatives'. The suggestion is that they only 'work' by sedating people with mental illnesses so they are necessarily 'less of a bother' to other people.

Behind this view there seems to lurk a moral argument, that using anything that sedates or is 'mind-altering' is (somehow) sinful. This logic is not, in my experience, spelled out, but the suggestion is made and left hanging in the air. It is true that if we are sedated we are less able to think clearly and act rationally, and so are more prone to sinful behaviour. But this also applies to non-drug-related situations.

As we saw earlier, when we have flu or have slept poorly, we are not mentally as alert. We are sedated like those who have taken drugs. In such circumstances we are more likely to sin because our self-control is impaired. When our children misbehave or the car breaks down, we are more likely to become irritated and speak morosely. The same is true if we use any of the many types of sedating medication, whether psychiatric or not. But this awareness should make us more careful to control ourselves. It is not an argument against medication any more than it is an argument against poor sleep or the flu. The implication of the language of 'mind-altering' is similarly that there is something fishy about these drugs. Again, though, people merely bad-mouth, without arguing a case.

Christian mind-altering

We do mind-altering every week in our church. We listen to God's word as it is taught and learn from it so that our understanding of his truth is improved and our thinking and behaviour are altered to be more like his. For we are to have our minds renewed through biblical teaching and so our behaviour changed too (Romans 12:2). It can, of course, be changed for bad if we conform to this world. This is why I find the 'mind-altering' innuendo peculiar. The real question is whether any alleged 'mind-altering' drugs cause us to think and do bad things, to sin. And for that there is no evidence at all.

But what about the purported risks from sedation? It is true that many psychiatric drugs are sedative. But others do the opposite, for they are alerting. This includes all the major anti-dementia drugs, such as those Malcolm received, methylphenidate (the most widely used drug in ADHD) and SSRIs (selective serotonin reuptake inhibitors, the most commonly prescribed type of antidepressants). But this sedation argument is a dangerous one to wield.

Those who argue we should avoid psychiatric drugs because they are sedative are likely to be hoisted by their own petard. A vast number of other widely prescribed drugs are also sedating, like commonly used painkillers such as co-codamol. This and other codeine-based analgesics can be bought over the counter without medical prescription and are used by large numbers of people with back-pain or headaches. Related opioid-based painkillers are given daily to large numbers of women in childbirth. Then, similarly, there are sedating treatments for urinary incontinence, epilepsy, hay fever and lots of other illnesses. If you claim it is wrong in principle to use psychiatric drugs merely because they are sedatives, then you will find you need to give up many, many medical treatments in order to be consistent. But actually there is direct biblical evidence supporting the use of 'mind-altering' and sedative substances.

Evidence from the vineyard

Psychiatric drugs are psychoactive, which roughly translated means 'mind-altering'. But the most widely used psychoactive drug in history is alcohol. In 1986 the Royal College of Psychiatrists published *Alcohol: Our Favourite Drug*, which discussed the risks and benefits of alcohol consumption. Alcohol acts as a molecule on receptors in the brain in the same way that prescribed drugs do. Psychiatric drugs, like painkillers, target the specific problem symptoms, such as hallucinations or pain, by modifying the chemicals in brain cells to treat these symptoms. Alcohol works in the same way.

Alcoholic drinks are referred to many times in the Scriptures. Most commonly this is to wine, but beer is often mentioned too (e.g. Leviticus 10:9; Numbers 6:3; Proverbs 20:1; and Luke 1:15). Wine is 'a fermented beverage made from the juice of grapes' and beer[6] is 'an intoxicating drink made from grain'.[7] In their lexicon Louw and Nida clarify,

> Though some . . . have argued that whenever mention is made of Jesus either making or drinking wine, one must assume that this was only unfermented grape juice, there is no real basis for such a conclusion. Only where *'oinos neos'* 'new wine' is mentioned can one assume that this is unfermented juice or grape juice in the initial stages of fermentation.[8]

It is clear that wine and beer were alcoholic beverages throughout the Old and New Testament periods. Otherwise why would drunkenness be a risk? See for example Genesis 9:21; Leviticus 10:9; Proverbs 23:30; Isaiah 28:7; and Ephesians 5:18. These alcohol-containing drinks were widely consumed as part of normal daily life in the ancient world. When commenting on the angelic prohibition (Luke 1:15) that John the Baptist was not to consume wine or beer, Joel Green states, 'Complete abstinence from wine and other alcoholic beverages is extraordinary in the biblical world, so the requirement that John embrace such ascetic behaviour requires explanation.'[9]

The positive mind-altering properties of wine are recognized, and commended, frequently in Scripture, for example, Judges 9:13; Psalm 104:15; Ecclesiastes 2:3; 9:7; 10:17; Song of Songs 1:2; 4:10; Isaiah 24:9; 25:6. Probably the most well known of these texts is Psalm 104:15, on which Calvin commented,

> In these words we are taught, that God not only provides
> for men's necessity, and bestows upon them as much as is
> sufficient for the ordinary purposes of life, but that in his
> goodness he deals still more bountifully with them by
> cheering their hearts with wine and oil. Nature would
> certainly be satisfied with water to drink; and therefore the
> addition of wine is owing to God's superabundant liberality.[10]

I agree with Calvin that the mind-altering ability of wine to relax us and make us feel better ('gladdens human hearts') is an aspect of God's goodness to us. But I would add that it also shows that using psychoactive drugs is legitimate, indeed can be good.

The straightjacket and the padded cell

It took Malcolm weeks to get better with his donepezil. While we waited, I sedated him with mild tranquillizers. The disturbed and aggressive behaviour of someone with psychosis will eventually respond to the drug's specific molecular properties. But what do we do in the meantime? Should we allow Malcolm to hurt himself and others by punching or kicking out in response to his hallucinations? Or is it better, as was done historically, to tie him up in a straightjacket? Or should we lock him up in a padded room? If it were true that it is morally wrong to use any drugs that sedate, then we would have to use the straightjacket instead. But we've seen from the Bible's teaching on alcohol that it is not wrong. The care of people with psychotic behaviour is extremely difficult. For those of us attempting to help, it is frustrating when others cast aspersions on effective medication without even suggesting alternatives.

ECT – it's Jack Nicholson's fault

Perhaps it would be fairer to blame Ken Kesey, who wrote *One Flew over the Cuckoo's Nest*, or the director of the film, Miloš Forman. But Jack Nicholson's performance in Hollywood's multiple-Oscar-winning misrepresentation of electroconvulsive therapy (ECT) in the film has a lot to answer for. It left the impression that ECT was a dangerous treatment that could fry the brains of unruly patients. I've looked down microscopes at brain tissue from patients who had lots of ECT, and it looks fine. But this film has left a terrible legacy to this day. While writing this book I've had a small part in a UK-wide clinical trial of ECT which attracted protests and an attempt to have it stopped by opponents. But before proceeding, we should place ECT in a wider medical context.

ECT involves passing an electric current through the brain in order to induce a convulsion (epileptic seizure). It is administered along with a muscle relaxant to modify the seizure and is carried out under a brief anaesthetic so the patient is unaware. Many randomized trials have established that it is a lot better than 'placebo' (here not a drug, but where individuals received only the anaesthetic but no ECT when unconscious). It is much better than antidepressants.[11] It is as effective in older people as it is in younger people, and it is safe in all age groups, during physical illness and in pregnancy.[12] ECT is especially effective in severe depression associated with psychosis, but it is also beneficial for other conditions too.[13]

Every day in every hospital doctors use knives to cut people open and chop out parts of their bodies (including brain tissue in neurosurgery). Yet such highly damaging surgical procedures don't attract the opprobrium of ECT. Doctors stick tubes into people's bowels, inject toxic drugs into their blood, or use radiation for tests that makes them more likely to get cancer. These and a host of other painful, dangerous and destructive procedures are carried out routinely all over the world without attracting the anger, political lobbying and hostile opposition that ECT does. It is difficult not to conclude that the stigma long associated with mental illness contributes to this double standard.

A miracle cure

The truth is that ECT is often the nearest thing we have to a miracle cure in psychiatry. Joan had lost several stone when I visited her urgently. My nursing colleague had grown very worried about her. Joan was experiencing auditory hallucinations and paranoid delusions (her neighbours were playing loud music to torment her and were planning on torturing her and killing her). She stopped her tablets. I had to bring her in to hospital urgently as it was clear she wasn't eating or drinking. I gave her urgent ECT. And a few weeks later she was well again. She had no hallucinations or delusions, and spoke warmly of her neighbours. She put on weight as she ate again and returned home.

Without ECT Joan might have died. Today it is easy to forget that some mental illnesses were fatal in the past, not via suicide (although that is clearly also sadly true), but by their direct morbid effects on the body. Even now some people with depression like Joan are so ill they can't eat and drink, and waste away. For them ECT is almost always curative and saves their lives.

Psychotherapy and counselling

It is helpful if we can distinguish counselling from the specific psychotherapies used in health services as treatments for mental illnesses. This is a bit difficult as the terms here are used loosely and so my headings are open to criticism. We will identify three categories.

First, there are specific (secular) psychotherapies that are based on a structured approach. Each is underpinned by a theoretical framework, which attempts to explain the mental illness. These formal psychotherapies require specialist training and are the 'talking treatments' used in psychiatric hospitals and clinics. There are a large number of such therapies, with new ones (or at least new variations) appearing from time to time.

Second, we have informal counselling. This is practised by Christian ministers and others in the church as part of their regular work. In this instance, it is based upon our biblical view of man and our salvation in Christ Jesus. It is also practised generally by psychiatrists, psychiatric nurses and others as part of their regular engagement with people with mental illnesses (although obviously without such a basis). Counselling like this is beneficial, as we saw when we looked at placebos. Shortly we'll look into how psychiatrists and Christian ministers can overlap and interact in this area.

Finally, for Christians, especially in the USA, there are various schools of 'Christian counselling' which offer services to help people with emotional problems and perhaps mental illnesses. These seem to fall somewhere in between these other two. They share with the specific (secular) psychotherapies a structured approach based upon models of human behaviour. The Christian counsellors and their schools use different models, which they try to build on a biblical view of humankind, in contrast to the secular psychotherapies.

But by constructing their models in this way they necessarily overlap with the informal counselling approach of Christian ministers. The latter may not have an explicit therapeutic model in mind, but ministers do have clear biblically informed views that may be very close to a structured model in practice. Unlike the specific secular psychotherapies, these Christian counselling approaches have not been tested in clinical trials. And so it is not clear whether they are more, or less, effective than the informal Christian counselling of ministers and mature Christians.

The failure of Freud

So let us look at specific (secular) psychotherapies. For much of the twentieth century Freudian psychotherapies claimed to be a panacea for all psychological and behavioural ills. But there was an elephant in the Freudian room: the absence of scientific evidence that they helped people. Dissenting voices dared to point to this elephant and ask why, if the claimed benefits were so great, there were no clinical trials to demonstrate this? In 1952 the academic psychiatrist, Professor Hans Eysenck, from the world-renowned Maudsley Hospital in London, published a controversial article reporting that only 44% of people improved with these treatments compared with 66% using other non-drug therapies (mainly behavioural therapies).[14] Freudians responded by claiming it was not possible to conduct randomized trials for psychotherapies.

Cognitive and behavioural therapies bury Freud

But the nails in the Freudian coffin were hammered home when other psychotherapies emerged which proved their benefits using randomized controlled trials. The first of these were behavioural therapies, such as those Eysenck designed. Such therapies have a limited range of use. They try to modify behaviours without regard to their underlying reasons.

Later cognitive therapy from Aaron Beck and others emerged. Today this is more usually known as cognitive-behavioural therapy (CBT) because it incorporates both cognitive (relating to thought processes) and behavioural elements. CBT encourages a collaborative approach between patient and therapist. Another type of psychotherapy with evidence of benefit is interpersonal therapy (IPT). IPT was another development in the later twentieth century. Like CBT, it is short-term and encourages the patient's 'ownership' of the illness-related problems. In IPT the focus is on relationships, and restoring these. These psychotherapies have been tested in different illnesses in randomized controlled trials and have proven their value.[15] Finally, under pressure to produce some evidence, trials of Freudian therapy were carried out . . . and they showed it didn't work.[16]

Cognitive-behavioural therapy (CBT)

CBT is the most widely used form of specialist psychotherapy. It was originally developed in the 1970s for depression. Later it was extended to anxiety, and more recently to other conditions, including schizophrenia and bipolar disorder. CBT is usually given to a single patient but it is also used for groups. In CBT there is a focus (as the name suggests) on both analysing the behaviours of the patient and on interpreting their thought processes accompanying these behaviours.

The CBT approach is collaborative, with the patient and therapist working closely together to agree on interpretations of their symptoms and on solutions. Patients are encouraged to work out their own solutions and to discuss their understanding of their illness symptoms with the therapist.

CBT characteristically focuses on the 'here and now' and not on the history and development of a mental illness. CBT theories are based on models of warped thinking patterns displayed by people with different kinds of mental illnesses. Patients are expected to take responsibility by doing 'homework' after each therapy session, in which they test out solutions for jointly identified key problems. A course of CBT is typically short-term, lasting twelve to sixteen sessions, once or twice a week. Helpful books from Christians explaining this approach are available.[17]

So CBT interpretations generally consider the current events and life context of the patient, with much less emphasis on the patient's past than other therapies. Of course, an understanding of the patient's earlier life experiences, and the views he or she has developed because of these, is often important. But CBT avoids attempts to delve around in the unconscious or to rake up past events unless something appears relevant.

In depression and anxiety, emotional states are understood to be fuelled by basic models of how the patients perceive themselves, the world around them and their future. When under stress, negative automatic thoughts emerge from these views which impact on mood. Thus a single young woman with depression, for example, may be struggling because her Christian worldview emphasizes the importance of marriage and children. Thus, when she interacts with men, she is unhelpfully and irrationally anxious and desiring to please. She repeatedly feels a failure when she does not find herself a partner.

Or an older man has filled his life with work and a successful career and then finds himself redundant. He generates negative thoughts whenever he meets people in work and despises himself as useless.

Be mindful about mindfulness

Riding the psychotherapy zeitgeist in the early twenty-first century is mindfulness. Its cultural status has been confirmed by it appearing twice this millennium on the front cover of *Time* magazine. But what exactly is it?

Two main types of mindfulness interventions have been used in healthcare: mindfulness-based cognitive therapy and mindfulness-based stress-reduction. Both are short-term, like CBT. And both involve melding techniques from established therapies on to Eastern mystical traditions. The essence of mindfulness is giving 'full attention to internal and external experiences as they occur in the present moment' and developing 'an attitude characterized by non-judgment of, and openness to, this current experience'.[18] In other words, you focus all your attention on some aspect of your current situation, viewing it from the outside without passing an opinion.

Does it work? Perhaps. Overall there is some evidence for modest benefit in depression, anxiety and various other illnesses.[19] But it is definitely not better than, and has much less evidence to support it, than CBT. Should Christians use it? The 2003 *Time* cover pictured a beautiful blonde woman in classic meditation pose. This is typical of mindfulness marketing. For although the medical therapies developed out of mindfulness may be employed devoid of their religious background, this is not the cultural perception.

If you used mindfulness, what message would you send? The 'weaker-brother principle' that Paul teaches in 1 Corinthians 8 and Romans 14 applies here, doesn't it? Paul warns Christians who have a better understanding of biblical truth (stronger ones) that they should be careful in exercising their mature grasp of Scripture in case they confuse less well-taught Christians (weaker ones). There is nothing wrong per se with relaxation techniques and quiet contemplation, although the non-judgmental element may be problematic if what is contemplated is immoral. But 'weaker brothers or sisters' who see you exercising this mature Christian freedom will conclude that Buddhism and Eastern mysticism generally can be integrated into Christianity, and they may be led into sin. So it is wiser to stick to CBT and other therapies which have no such religious associations.

How good are psychiatric treatments?

Critics of antidepressants, and other psychiatric drugs, have used the scientifically proven small benefit achieved by the former to claim they are not much good. And since they have side effects, they are best avoided. If this claim were true for antidepressants, then, applying the same logic, they would also have to apply it to CBT. (Yes, CBT has side effects! See below.) And even more so to other psychotherapies for which evidence is much weaker. In fact, the claims for antidepressants are based on a much larger number of trials and a much larger number of subjects.[20]

But I don't think the claim is true in either case. Both CBT and antidepressants are safe and effective. Back to Malcolm. Remember, he would never have entered a drug trial. Or any kind of trial. Clinical trials prove that treatments work. But they don't tell us how much they work. This is partly because they were not designed for this (another story), and partly because they don't include the sickest people. We know that the sicker people are in these studies, the more they benefit. And so the sickest people like Malcolm would have much larger benefits if they could be studied in trials. But they can't.

And there is another reason why treatments don't work well sometimes. People simply don't use them. In research trials a lot of patients don't take all their tablets or complete their CBT. In one schizophrenia study I worked on a third of patients stopped taking their drugs (probably more; a third actually told us they had). There are good reasons (again a long story) for including everyone when we work out how effective a treatment is overall. And so in this study the drug was very effective overall for schizophrenia, even including the third of people who didn't take it! But when patients take drugs we see even better benefits.

Sometimes when teaching on treatments, I'm asked by other doctors why we see such small benefits in research studies compared with what we all experience in our clinics. Now you know why.

First do no harm

The media would have you believe that talking therapies do no harm. They are a kind of wonder treatment that has only benefits and no side effects. But the idea that drugs have harms and 'talking treatments' don't is nonsense. It has been recognized and reported for decades that psychotherapies can harm you. Therapists themselves report adverse effects in about 10% of people and have called for better research to help us understand this.[21] After all, if any treatment is powerful enough to help and heal, then it is powerful enough also to harm.

Megan had depression with marked anxiety. She was referred by a colleague to receive psychotherapy. I was summoned urgently to see her in clinic where she was screaming in distress and saying she wanted to go home and kill herself. Her (inexperienced) therapist had provoked this reaction by insensitively discussing abuse-related matters, and she had to be admitted to hospital. If she had been in a drug trial, this would have been classed as a severe adverse reaction and she would never receive the drug again. Incredibly, the therapist wanted her to resume therapy after leaving hospital. Sadly, even some therapists don't acknowledge that their treatments can harm.

Rarely discussed is the risk of sexual abuse of patients by therapists. The set-up in psychotherapy is one in which biblically minded Christians, indeed anyone with common sense, will see an obvious risk of this happening. A powerful professional figure spends long periods alone with a vulnerable patient. Christian ministers, and others conducting pastoral visits, will wish to avoid this sort of situation lest they are tempted into inappropriate sexual conduct. A survey in the USA reported that 7% of male and 3% of female psychotherapists had engaged in sexual contact with their patients.[22]

The eminent British psychiatrist Professor David Nutt, of University College London, has reported this to be more likely, unsurprisingly, during the longer-term Freudian psychotherapies. Based on GMC (General Medical Council, the UK regulatory body for medical practitioners) data, Nutt estimated that the risk of sexual abuse is at least three cases per 100,000 contacts (likely to be much higher since this is based only on doctors and only on reported cases). A drug treatment with this frequency of severe side effects would be likely to be refused a prescribing licence by regulators.[23]

Of course drugs harm too. If you read the insert with any drug (the tightly folded sheet of paper), it lists a large number of side effects. For licensed treatments serious risks are rare, otherwise they wouldn't have been licensed in the first place. But they are real and need to be balanced against the potential benefits. I think antidepressants are overprescribed, often given for mild depression (or no depressive illness at all) where the risks of harm outweigh the benefits. It is recognized that antipsychotic drugs were overprescribed in dementia for many years. Research I was involved in helped recognize this and prompted a welcome huge reduction in their use. Likewise, the real benefits and the potential harms of psychotherapies need to be weighed up for each person.

Christian informal counselling

Every time psychiatrists meet a patient they should be carefully questioning and listening sympathetically to learn what they need to know in order to make a diagnosis and inform their care (what we call 'management'). And they should also be warmly and intelligently engaging with patients like this to understand their specific difficulties and distress. We've seen that such engagement is therapeutic and is sometimes referred to as 'informal counselling'. It is similar to the kind of informal support and advice people give one another every day. Sometimes we make off-the-cuff remarks based on our own experience. At other times it may be more planned, when someone comes to ask for advice. But we know some people are better at this than others, and the Bible gives us a couple of reasons why.

Wisdom

When I was a child, I used to think some older people were very clever. They made me feel rather dim. Walking through a local wood as a boy, I came to a gate that was stuck. I pushed and pulled and couldn't open it. Then an old man arrived. He put his foot under the gate, gently lifted it and released the gate – brilliant, so clever! Except that he had been there before. My vanity tells me that previously he had pushed and pulled too! Experience brings such wisdom in everyday life. We may call this skill.

Experience helps in the realm of moral behaviour and counselling too. But here the Bible teaches us we also need a proper attitude to the Lord. We need a holy fear of him so that we live each moment aware of his presence, constantly seeking to make decisions that are right in his sight. Such wisdom grows and is refined by experience and so is generally related to age. But not automatically.

In the book of Proverbs the wise are those who listen and observe and learn. They are keen to seek advice and to take it. The foolish are the opposite. They are sluggards who don't make the effort to seek advice and learn. When talking with a minister about such matters some years ago at a meeting, he gestured to a couple of other ministers nearby. He commented that one, in his twenties, had already become a wise, mature servant of Christ in his church. But the other older man had, he declared, learnt nothing in twenty years (he was too kind to call him a fool).

Giftedness

Whether psychotherapy is specific or supportive, secular or Christian, its success is strongly related to the personal qualities of the counsellor. Some people are simply better at it. They have good people skills. Or as the Scriptures teach, some are more gifted than others. They are better listeners, more shrewd at weighing what they hear, more emotionally engaging, more empathic and so on. So while every minister should have the biblically informed wisdom to counsel people in distress, others in the church may be better equipped to do so.

Such people should also be mature, wise and have a sound knowledge of scriptural teaching. But they are also blessed with superior interpersonal skills and so are better equipped to counsel and help others. Every church should seek to identify those men and women who have these attributes so they can be called upon to help as the need arises. In good churches this will already be happening. Church leaders will know who are best equipped to counsel and who can be called upon to support and guide others in their distress.

Working with the psychiatrist

Christian leaders should be thoroughly grounded in biblical teaching, mature in Christ, and thus wise. So when a young man (Josh) visits to discuss how he should conduct himself with his fiancée, and expresses concern about his struggles with the temptation to sexual sin, a Christian leader is able to offer sound advice.

But what if Josh is also hallucinating? What if alongside this relationship issue he asks about 'the voices'? Is a church leader now competent to counsel him? Yes and no. He (man to man is wisest for this situation) is just as able to impart his biblical wisdom on his relationship with his fiancée. And he can express understanding and sympathy for his plight. He may counsel Josh on how to respond to the hallucinations if they are suggesting immoral behaviour. But he will also recognize that Josh is ill and needs medical help too.

So what about the psychiatrist? He (or she) too should have developed wisdom in the biblical sense of 'skill'. His skill will be like that of the minister in questioning, listening and understanding how people tick. His years of clinical work should have finely tuned his ability to interpret people. And his specific training in mental illness will have enabled him to interpret the key symptoms of mental illnesses so he makes accurate diagnoses. He will determine whether Josh has auditory hallucinations and may conclude he has acute schizophrenia. He may recommend antipsychotic medication and a course of CBT to help him handle his symptoms more effectively.

But with regard to Josh's relationship with his fiancée, then the psychiatrist's advice will be determined by what he thinks best for his illness. He may conclude that the comfort and support of this relationship with his fiancée, including the sex, will be beneficial to his recovery, and advise accordingly. Or he may think that the emotional stress of conducting the relationship may worsen his illness, and so counsel a period of separation.

The psychiatrist will give advice related to the illness and generally avoid moral counsel. If Josh tells him he is an evangelical Christian and that sex outside marriage is wrong, the psychiatrist is unlikely to argue otherwise. However, he may do so if he thinks this would be best for him. This is why it is important for his minister, or other church leader, to be involved. Most of the time counsel from a psychiatrist (or others such as a psychologist or a nurse) will be pragmatic and avoid moral issues. But this is far from guaranteed. Hence the importance of support from people in Josh's church.

If, like me, the psychiatrist is a Christian, then ideally his counsel should be the same as that of the minister. I say 'ideally' not because the Christian psychiatrist and minister might differ in biblical interpretation (which is clearly quite possible), but because the minister is actually much better placed to counsel Josh than his psychiatrist. The minister will almost certainly know Josh much better. He will know the key details of his life and the kind of relationships he has with his family and friends at church. We know that the details, the nitty-gritty, of wise advice are crucial to effective counsel or therapy. And that established relationships can buffer the impact of mental illness and support Josh in his recovery.

So Josh's minister should be able to counsel him sensitively and carefully on his relationship with his fiancée, and encourage him in a righteous pattern of behaviour. His psychiatrist should be able to assess him thoroughly, make a correct diagnosis and implement effective medical treatment. The psychiatrist and the minister have complementary and overlapping roles.

Key chapter points

- We are blessed with many very effective and safe drug treatments.
- ECT is safe and one of the most effective treatments in medicine.

- CBT and related psychotherapies are of established benefit in milder illnesses and complement medication in more severe illnesses.
- The knowledge and experience of church leaders and their established relationships with church members make them very well placed to help people effectively with mental illnesses.
- Church leaders have a complementary role to specialists in psychiatry, which enhances the overall quality of care for people with mental illnesses.

8. PSYCHOSOMATIC ILLNESSES

'Are you a hawk or a dove?' is a question often asked during the summer examinations period when we examiners gather at the medical school. I try to avoid answering, stating that I cannot judge myself, but some people are keen to tell me that I am a dove, while others regard me as a hawk. Since the medical school has recently started comparing marks from all examiners, there is now a definitive answer! Hawks are hardliners, those who seek out mistakes and, in clinical exams, ask especially difficult questions to expose the weaknesses of students. Doves are more generous in their approach, keen to be supportive and encouraging and ask more straightforward questions.

Are you a hawk or a dove when it comes to people with psychosomatic illnesses? When reading the material on hysteria and shell shock in chapter 5, did you find yourself criticizing the people with these conditions, suspecting these were not real illnesses? Or did you adopt a more dovish approach, seeing them as people in need of help, suffering people for whom you felt sympathy?

And what about other conditions which remain charged issues? Are you a hawk or a dove when it comes to chronic fatigue syndrome, fibromyalgia or irritable bowel syndrome? These are modern conditions on the fringe of psychiatry. Do you feel hawkish towards people with anxiety disorders, such as agoraphobia or obsessive-compulsive disorder? Are you dovish when you meet someone with anorexia nervosa? These eating disorders were once part of hysteria.[1] This group of people is characterized by a bewildering range of fluctuating symptoms, such as fatigue, aches and pains, faints, fits, dizziness, anxiety, depressed moods, eating problems and emotional lability. They frequently attend GP practices and commonly seek help from church leaders.

In this book I am calling these conditions 'psychosomatic', but the equally broad label of 'neurosis' could also be used. Historically, both have been labelled this way.[2] I prefer the term 'psychosomatic' because it corresponds to our human nature as body and soul, reminding us of this important truth. And it reminds us too that these conditions all have a complex mix of mental and physical symptoms.

Frauds, distressed or sick?

Are such people sick? Professor of Psychiatry Simon Wessely, comments, 'The passions that these arguments create are because what is at stake is the issue of legitimacy – what constitutes an acceptable disease, and what is legitimate suffering worthy of support and sympathy?'[3] Philosopher Ian Hacking observes,

> We are besieged by mental illnesses, more neurotic than psychotic, and we wonder which of them are affectations, cultural artifacts, clinician enhanced, or copycat syndromes,

and which ones are, as we briefly and obscurely put it, real. We are profoundly confused about an entire group of mental disorders, feeling that their symptoms are both nurtured and natural, both moral and neurological.[4]

Multiple boundaries

The reader will guess that this subheading refers not to the latest explosive batting from Alex Hales or Ben Stokes, but to how we understand the relationship of these psychosomatic mental illnesses to other conditions. Psychosomatic illnesses fit our definition of mental illness. They lead to significant and disabling impairments in daily living and result from objective events. They are real illnesses. But ones in which drawing the line is especially tricky. Recognizing this, we should take a dovish approach to such people, and not be inclined to suspicion.

We've seen that there is no clear boundary between these psychosomatic illnesses and normal distress. There is also no clear boundary between these and what are generally regarded as physical illnesses. As a society, we are confused also about a distinction between psychosomatic illnesses which are regarded as physical illnesses (e.g. fibromyalgia and irritable bowel syndrome) and those which are regarded as mental illnesses (such as anorexia nervosa and generalized anxiety disorder). They share fluctuating emotionally driven symptoms involving mind and body.

But, for this chapter, it is the absence of clear boundaries between the different psychosomatic illnesses that is most relevant. Does that statement make sense? Perhaps not. How can you have boundaries if there not different things to separate? What I mean is that a lot of diagnoses shelter under this big umbrella and overlap with one another. Obsessive-compulsive disorder (OCD), generalized anxiety disorder

(GAD), anorexia nervosa and post-traumatic stress disorder (PTSD) are some of the most well known. But in our current state of knowledge it is far from clear that any of these individual labels are meaningfully describing separate entities. Historically, they were lumped together, and over time people change from one to another.

Their symptoms are driven by mood changes (anxiety and depression symptoms). Treatment for all should be holistic, involving physical and psychological approaches. The severe mental illnesses of the next chapter will also require both physical and psychological treatments, but the physical and psychological treatments we employ will vary with those different illnesses. Here they are much the same. Hence it is preferable that we deal with them together. Below in the patient examples I will use the standard current diagnoses for convenience and ease of communication, not because they are well-defined entities.

Helping people with psychosomatic illnesses: stepped care

Stepped care refers to a graded approach to treatment and is employed widely in psychiatry and medicine. It is important here because the early steps do not require specialist expertise. They can be used by church leaders, resulting in real benefits for sufferers in our churches.[5] Some people with more complex and severe illnesses may need help delivered by those with specialist experience. But for most patients with psychosomatic illnesses, and for those with stress-related problems not crossing the illness boundary, church leaders can help people apply the following steps. Those with milder illnesses can be treated with a judicious combination of these steps and additional specific medical treatments.

1. Supportive relationships[6]

The essential context for effective medical treatment is a good relationship, just as it is for effective pastoral ministry. This fits with what we saw in chapter 2 about our image-ness: we were created to be in relationships. But it takes two. A relationship involves commitment from both parties. A major cause of failure of medical treatment is lack of engagement. And the same is true in pastoring, isn't it? A major reason why people don't respond to help from church leaders is a lack of commitment. With no meaningful relationship, little progress can be made. All the other elements of stepped care below depend upon a good relationship, with both parties committed to the patient getting better.

This is not intended to shift the blame for failure on to the patient. It takes two. I need to work from my side to engage and establish a warm, trusting relationship. And with the mentally ill I need to work especially hard, because, as we've seen, they are damaged in their ability to form and maintain such relationships. Kindness and perseverance will commonly be needed to form such good relationships. But the good news is that church leaders usually have a head start here. At work I have to start from scratch in getting to know someone and this can take a long time. In the church relationships are already established. I made this important point earlier: church leaders are very well placed to support and help the mentally ill.

Within the context of such relationships, church leaders can exercise their wisdom and personal skills to help the afflicted. Getting the basics right is vital. You don't become a skilled pianist without arduous practice learning the scales, you don't become a good footballer without long hours at the training ground mastering core skills, and you don't help people with mental illness without deliberate effort to establish and maintain good relationships.

2. Meaningful work

Discussion on the fourth commandment often misses the fact that this includes a command to work. We are to enjoy a balanced week of six days of work and one day of worship. We saw in chapter 2 that we were created to 'work', that is, to carry out the cultural mandate of ruling the earth under God. This work is not synonymous with paid employment, but includes all kinds of scientific, artistic and technological endeavours, whether pursued with our hands or our heads. It is good and healthy.

Of course, in this fallen world work is often painful and hard, and work can be a place where stress contributes to mental illness. But 'meaningful work', activity that is pleasurable and fulfilling, pushes in the opposite direction. It can help to heal and is an important part of the whole healing context. We should aim to help people find as much good and enjoyable working activity as we can. This is important mentally in providing contentment and pleasure, which combat the anxiety and depressive symptoms of psychosomatic illnesses.

Work is also important because it provides structure and routine. God is a God of order, and we, as image-bearers, are meant to imitate him in this. The weekly pattern is part of this. Daily and weekly and annual patterns of living were integral to how Israel was told to live in the Old Testament. These are good for us. Routine provides stability, while the loss of routine breeds stress with its associated sadness and anxiety.

Many people with psychosomatic illnesses are not living with such a 'work–life balance'. They have lost these regular habits and rhythms and perhaps lost meaningful work. We should encourage them to restore such habits if they have been lost. Or if they have never established such habits, we help them figure out how to do so.

3. Diet and exercise

I can hear many in my own church laughing at the above heading. Those who know me would smile at the idea that I am advocating a healthy diet! There is a keen allotment owner in my church who grows prodigious quantities of green vegetables and brings lots of these to give away. Now, I like fruit and other vegetables, just not these ones. And I don't like the 'five-a-day' mantra because it is dogma without evidence. But that is the scientist in me quibbling. Regular moderate exercise and a balanced diet should fit into our daily and weekly routine. Regular moderate exercise is good for mind and body. One of the reasons for the great improvement in health in the UK over the past century has been a healthier lifestyle, with better diet being central to this. And this seems to have applied to mental illnesses too, including schizophrenia and dementia.[7]

4. Substance avoidance

'Legal highs' and illicit drugs don't help mental illness, but the long-standing legal substances – nicotine, alcohol and caffeine – can all precipitate and worsen anxiety too. They do so when taken in excess or when we withdraw from their (excessive) use. Alcohol and smoking are often used as 'self-medication' to treat anxiety and low mood. And so are illegal substances such as cannabis, which are widely available. I'm sure their use is less of a problem in churches than outside, although I'm not sure there is data to support this assertion. But we are blind if we pretend that their misuse doesn't happen. Within the context of a good relationship, careful, sensitive exploration of the use of these substances is important. And it can be very tricky.

Liz did very well on antidepressants and got almost well. But she was left with disabling and fluctuating anxiety. Fiddling with medication didn't solve it. Neither did CBT. Liz repeatedly denied any misuse of alcohol or anything else. Then one day a shrewd community nurse popped in unannounced and found the bottles of wine. We thought we had a good relationship with Liz. Perhaps we did. Just not quite good enough to enable her to overcome her shame. Once it was out in the open, she was able to deal with it, control her drinking, and get well and back to regular work.

Andy was under pressure at work. He needed to deliver his project and the deadline rushed upon him. He wasn't sleeping and felt tense and irritable all day long. A colleague suggested he should see his GP. Andy reluctantly agreed, and after a chat and physical work-up, his GP reassured him there was nothing to worry about. His pastor Bob wasn't quite so sure. He had watched Andy disappear quickly from church meetings and then stop attending. He knew he was working very long hours. When he visited, he found Andy beavering away in the evening, consuming strong coffee. He learned that Andy was drinking 'maybe thirty mugs a day'. He said it wasn't surprising he couldn't sleep and persuaded him to cut back to his previous four to five mugs. He also worked with Andy to schedule regular breaks, including ensuring a return to services where he would enjoy meeting his church friends again. Andy's anxiety settled, his work productivity improved and he completed his project on time. Andy's good relationship with Bob, and Bob's knowledge of Andy's lifestyle, enabled them to work it out.

5. Sleep hygiene

Perhaps you didn't know you could have unhygienic sleep? You can mess up your sleep by going to bed at irregular times; getting up irregularly; catnapping by day; not exercising;

drinking coffee or tea or alcohol shortly before going to bed; and taking your smartphone to bed with you. Oh, and of course you can ensure the bedroom is noisy and light and the bed is uncomfortable. Few people manage to tick all of these, but even a few of them can disturb sleep quality, which lowers mood and worsens anxiety.

Once again there are simple steps to take here which can make small but important differences. You don't need to be a doctor or sleep specialist. There is more to it, of course, but getting these basics right helps. It is not difficult in theory; in practice, it is often very difficult. People are bonded to their phones nowadays, and many, especially those with mental illnesses, have developed erratic living patterns that need to be gently corrected.

So here is a structured approach. As a friend commented, it is largely a case of 'following the Maker's instructions'. But many people, especially those with mental illnesses, struggle to do this, and helping them to do so can lead to substantial benefit.

Specific medical treatments

While church leaders and churches can provide this important context to facilitate the healing of people with psychosomatic illnesses, health services will implement specific treatments. We've seen how our psychosomatic nature means that both physical and psychological components are required in therapy, and this is especially true of these psychosomatic illnesses. In health services this can be difficult. Many patients are convinced that there must be a physical cure. If I had a pound for every patient who wanted me to cure them with a tablet, I wouldn't quite be a very rich man but I would have acquired a tidy sum of money. Yet for individuals with these illnesses it is psychological therapies that are usually most helpful.

Psychological approaches

All the guidelines say that psychological approaches should be carried out first. For milder illnesses, such help should be sought out, and much good can be done by church leaders, as discussed in the previous chapter. In practice, pragmatically medication is often used first due to time pressure and the patchy availability of psychotherapies. For milder conditions, psychological approaches delivered in primary-care settings should be sufficient, and secondary care psychiatry involvement is not necessary.[8] For people with moderate to severe illnesses, medication becomes necessary, at least in the short term, with psychotherapies continuing to have a key role.

Psychoeducation

GPs and healthcare professionals in specialist services will provide some kind of education and information about the patient's problems. Gaining an understanding of how the different symptoms relate to one another is helpful, for example that low mood makes pain worse, and so treating this can help with pain control. And many people are worried that their physical symptoms are features of some terrible, perhaps fatal, disease. Judicious medical assessment and investigation can help deal with such fears and relieve this anxiety and related symptoms. Of course, for some people the fact that a doctor decides to 'just do some tests' might confirm their worst fears, since 'they wouldn't do this unless they thought I had cancer, would they?' Again, knowing the person is vital to making the correct decision here.

Specific psychological therapies

There are a lot of different names given to very similar psycho-therapies, and the therapy used is likely to be determined by local availability. Relaxation training can be generally helpful, and alongside psychoeducation may be all that is needed for some who are well supported and utilizing the above earlier steps of care.

Behavioural treatments can be helpful for anxiety related to phobias or for compulsive rituals in OCD or for eating problems. Since psychosomatic illnesses have prominent mood symptoms that worsen the physical symptoms, then much of the focus is on relieving these mood changes. This is beneficial in itself, but has knock-on benefits for other symptoms too. Variants of CBT, such as problem-solving therapy and anxiety management, focus on specific problem areas. Their focus helps make them simpler and so more widely available. Fuller CBT may be employed for the whole range of psychosomatic conditions. Church leaders can learn to use some CBT techniques to manage low mood and anxiety in people with milder conditions.[9]

Medication

The two main types of drug used for these illnesses are benzodiazepines and antidepressants. Benzodiazepines (e.g. diazepam (Valium)) are misleadingly called minor tranquil-lizers. They are actually quite powerful and are used as anaesthetics for minor procedures! They have several import-ant properties and the key one here is that they act at specific brain receptors to relieve anxiety. They are very effective anti-anxiety drugs. Arguably too effective! People easily become addicted to them. This leads to dependence, and then the anti-anxiety benefits also disappear. They can be helpful in times of severe anxiety-driven distress, but should only be used for a few weeks while psychological treatments are initiated. In addition to leading to dependence, they have important side effects. They can make people unsteady on their feet and prone to fall, especially older people.

Antidepressants are discussed in chapter 9. They are of proven benefit for obsessions and compulsions and some severe anxiety with panic attacks. They have the advantage that they can be used safely in the long term without dependence, but such long-term use should be restricted to the minority of people who have more severe illnesses.

Clinical case examples

The examples below illustrate the most common types of psychosomatic illness and the standard diagnoses applied today. My reservations about the scientific underpinning of these specific diagnoses are clear, but I recognize the value of having labels that help communicate the patterns of illness symptoms people experience.

Jim (generalized anxiety disorder with tension headache)

Jim was a teacher who developed bad headaches. He had grown very tired at school, feeling tense and worrying about his work, especially the upcoming assembly. When anxious, he noticed his heart pounding and sometimes he had tingling feelings in his arms and legs. His anxiety had grown worse because he felt he had flunked the previous assembly and would do so again.

He had been anxious for years at work. It had just got worse since that dreadful assembly. His headaches became so bad that he was laid up in bed and couldn't get to work. His GP visited and couldn't find any physical problem. He encouraged Jim to take paracetamol. His headache settled a little and after several days he recovered enough to get back to his teaching. On his return, a friend jested about how Jim had managed to escape taking the school assembly. Jim continued to be tense and tired and often struggled to concentrate enough to teach his classes. But he just about coped. Until the school sports day.

As this approached, with all the extra duties and responsibility, his headache returned. Again he was off sick and so missed the sports day. On his return, he was asked to see his head teacher, who suggested he see his GP as he was clearly struggling. He saw a different doctor who gave more time and identified these key elements in Jim's illness. This doctor recognized that Jim's headache was related to his generalized anxiety, which was long-standing, and arranged for him to see a community nurse for anxiety management. The doctor also encouraged Jim to be candid with his head teacher about his fears when taking the assembly or sports day duties. His head agreed it would be best to relieve him of all such extra responsibilities. With this, and with the anxiety management, his tension, worries and other symptoms improved and he coped at work.

For people like Jim, the temptation for a doctor is to prescribe drugs. But they do not help. Church leaders can use the stepped-care approach above and elements of anxiety management, and these may be enough for many people. For others, some specialist help like Jim received will be required.

Mani (anorexia nervosa[10])

Mani was a young woman at a sixth form college who appeared generally content and well engaged. She enjoyed good relationships with her family and at church. But one day Fiona, the minister's wife, received a call from Mani's mother expressing concern about her health. She had lost a lot of weight, stopped menstruating and done surprisingly poorly in her recent essays. Fiona knew Mani well from their youth group days and, after checking that Mani was aware her mother had spoken to her, Fiona was able to meet with her.

Mani admitted she had been eating less and less because she was worried she had become fat: her account suggested she was eating virtually nothing. Fiona suggested Mani looked rather thin, but Mani insisted she was overweight with very fat legs. She acknowledged she was doing more running and cycling than ever so that she would lose weight. She admitted she felt miserable whenever she remembered 'friends' at school who had called her fat. She struggled to concentrate when doing her studies at home and at the college campus. She believed that others, especially young men, perceived her to be 'fat and ugly'.

Fiona also spoke with Mani's mother, who admitted she had thought all this dieting and exercise would be just a passing fad. Shopping and cooking had become very difficult because Mani obsessionally watched the calories of everything and carefully measured her portion sizes. She had, for example, checked the calories in every brand of yogurt and insisted she would only eat Asda's own brand because these had slightly fewer calories than others.

Fiona and her mother arranged for Mani to meet regularly with Fiona and persuaded her to see her GP, who found her blood tests all to be normal, but her weight to be abnormally low with a body mass index (BMI) of 16.6.[11] It was clear that it was her desire to become thin and beautiful that had been driving her behaviour, and that she had anorexia nervosa. The GP helped Mani admit she needed to change her lifestyle, gave her information on anorexia nervosa and arranged for her to see a dietician to draw up a more reasonable healthy diet.

Mani agreed to work towards a target BMI of 20 and to discuss this and her revised diet with her mother.

Fiona discussed the cultural pressures pushing young women towards abnormal thinness and unattainable ideals of physical beauty. She emphasized that beauty is about far more than physical appearance, and successful marriages are largely about healthy relationships. She reassured Mani that she was a lovely young woman who was liked and respected in the church and by her parents. Mani's parents patiently encouraged Mani to stick to her new diet and reduced exercise schedule, and helped her to unload about pressures at the college. With such family and church support, Mani reached her target weight, began menstruating again and achieved good A level results at the end of college.

Mani's anorexia was mild, but in some people anorexia can be life-threatening and require inpatient care in hospital. But most cases are nearer to normality like Mani's and to the widespread dieting and thinness behaviours of young (and not so young) women. Although usually a condition of young women, it does also occur in men and in older adults. For those with milder problems (which may or may not cross the line into illness), sympathetic and candid discussion and simple supportive plans, for example monitoring of diet and restriction of time exercising, will be sufficient. If such approaches are not successful, or in more advanced cases where engagement and discussion are difficult, then the involvement of medical and psychiatric services will be required. However, as always, the continuing support of the church, as well as family, is important to a successful recovery.

Marjorie (mixed anxiety and depression)
Marjorie was a long-standing member of the church, but a 'high-maintenance' one for her minister. Her GPs regarded

her as 'a heart-sink patient'. Her past had always been difficult to clarify due to her marked tendency to embellish lavishly all descriptions about her life. It seemed clear that her childhood had been hard, and may have involved physical and perhaps sexual abuse. She had lost contact with her parents and siblings many years before in her late teens when she had moved away from her home town.

She came into contact with the church, attended outreach meetings and Christianity Explored home groups and was converted and baptized. She had been a regular since and had slowly grown in her understanding of the faith. But she also suffered bouts of significant anxiety and distress during which she withdrew from the church. On such occasions her minister would find her weepy and complaining of various ailments for which her GP could find no cause. Sometimes she has also been off work during such episodes and has seen psychiatrists who prescribed antidepressants. She told her minister that she was 'a mystery to doctors'. Over the years they had diagnosed her with 'depression', 'generalized anxiety disorder', 'tension headache', 'irritable bowel syndrome' and 'somatization disorder'.

Marjorie's minister did not need to worry about the medical diagnosis. She had a psychosomatic illness with its character-istic fluctuating pattern of symptoms. Medication doesn't help such people. But the above stepped approach can, perhaps combined with a psychotherapy. Whether or not she needed to see her GP or a psychiatrist on any particular occasion, she would always benefit from the personal wisdom and guidance that mature Christian leaders can give. And from the practical help and comfort from visits from church members. The value of such 'simple' measures should not be missed for such fragile people, regardless of whether mental illness is, or is not, present.

Graham (obsessive-compulsive disorder (OCD) and mild depression)

Kath knew Graham had always been a careful and tidy person. She had appreciated the way he kept their home, but over several months she thought he had 'lost the plot'. Whenever they went out, it took him an hour or more to get ready. He would walk endlessly around the house checking the locks and making sure all the appliances and electric sockets were switched off. Round and round he went – kettle, toaster, microwave, kitchen door, lamp, TV, front door, back door, kettle, toaster and so on. The final straw was when these checking rituals moved upstairs too and delayed Kath getting to bed.

Whenever she discussed it, he spoke about the fire safety course at work, with its warnings about how fires can start from appliances left on overnight. And he reminded her about the TV crime programmes highlighting the risks of burglary. 'But why do you need to check everything ten times?' Kath would ask in despair. Graham needed to do these rituals to quash his anxiety. If he didn't, he felt a horrid painful discomfort. Performing his checking rituals would alleviate this. At first, to calm himself, he had only needed to do everything twice, but it had grown to ten times. And now everything had to be checked in exactly the same sequence. If he was distracted and got the order wrong (or more likely worried he had done so), he had to start all over again. Only the correct sequence would do.

Kath also noticed that he had become more gloomy and irritable. He complained often of being tired and he had lost all interest in sex. He found it difficult to concentrate at work and had been warned by his boss about his performance. His thoughts were consumed by fears of burglary and fire if he failed to complete his sequences properly. Meals were delayed and his relationship with Kath became strained. When his rituals began keeping her up very late at night, she finally discussed it with Doreen at church.

Doreen laughed at first: 'We all worry about that . . . and everyone checks their locks, don't they?' But when Doreen asked a bit more carefully, she became concerned as well. Everyone did not check ten times. No-one she knew felt compelled to do it in exactly the same sequence. And she had noticed Graham had become withdrawn at church too. She mentioned the problem to their minister, Trevor, who agreed it was a concern.

Trevor spent some time meeting with Graham to under-stand the situation better and advise him. Graham confided that he hadn't told Kath about his 'great sin'. At work he had failed to speak up when colleagues blasphemed. Since then he had experienced repeated thoughts about denying Jesus. To counter these he kept repeating, 'I will not deny my Lord.' He had become convinced that if he repeated this ten times every time he thought of denying Jesus, then he would be all right.

Trevor could see that all this was way beyond normal worrying. He suggested Graham visit his GP while Doreen met up with Kath to support her. Graham's GP thought he had become depressed, but in an unusual way. He started him on the antidepressant citalopram and referred him to the local psychiatry service. The psychiatrist identified his repeated religious thoughts as obsessional ones that Graham was neutralizing using a covert thought ritual (repeating 'I will not deny my Lord') and explained his checking behaviour as a compulsive ritual to counteract his anxiety. This had all been brought on by a mild depressive illness. The psychiatrist arranged for CBT and increased his dose of citalopram. Graham recovered over the following months with such combined treatment and continuing support from Trevor.

OCD is commonly associated with depression, and obsessional symptoms frequently occur in other psychosomatic illnesses. Like Graham, people with OCD don't just have more frequent repeated thoughts (obsessions) and repetitive behaviours (rituals). They suffer intense and increasing anxiety, which they believe they can control only by carrying out rituals. These may be mental (repeating statements like Graham's) or compulsive behaviours (such as repeated cleaning, washing or checking). These rituals temporarily alleviate the painful anxiety. Most people with OCD benefit from selective serotonin reuptake inhibitor (SSRI) medication, and CBT is usually helpful too. A small proportion have more severe OCD, which requires longer-term engagement with psychiatric services.

Sophie (fibromyalgia[12] and low mood)

Sophie had persistent pain in several muscles in her arms and legs, poor sleep and fatigue. Medical investigations did not yield evidence of a clear cause. She was diagnosed with fibromyalgia by a hospital specialist. Painkillers provided some help, but her GP took a wider view. She noticed that her fibromyalgia had begun with a severe viral illness. But also that Sophie and her husband Raj had already had marital problems, with the associated distress. These difficulties had been eased when her husband Raj had taken on the caring role of looking after her. Furthermore, there was stress at work where Sophie felt she had been performing poorly, and so she had become 'depressed' at this perceived failure.

Her family had always ridiculed psychiatry, claiming that only the weak and feeble develop 'so-called mental illnesses'. The GP recognized that Sophie's fibromyalgia was closely related to these personal problems at home and at work. She arranged a series of sessions of CBT that focused on her mood and related physical symptoms. The GP also met Raj and encouraged him to withdraw gradually from his supportive role, and to re-engage with Sophie in a normal way as a husband rather than as a carer. The painkillers were continued, but with this multifaceted approach she recovered and returned to work.

Failure to identify any clear cause of pain, fatigue, headache and other physical symptoms is common. Sometimes this may reflect our medical ignorance, but even when a potential physical cause, for example osteoarthritis, can be identified, the psychological component is usually important, as with Sophie. An irony of the reluctance of some doctors and patients to recognize the role of such mental factors is that they are quite treatable. Even where we seem to have no specific treatment for the physical problem, we can, through the application of the simple stepped-care approach and skilled use of psychological treatments, provide meaningful help.

Helen (agoraphobia)

Helen was taking her usual bus to the office when she began to feel overheated and panicky. Her anxiety escalated into a panic attack during which she believed she was about to die of a heart attack. She got off the bus at the next stop and took a taxi home. She slept badly that night, and when she woke up was filled with dread about getting on the bus. She felt her heart racing again, knew she was over-breathing (hyperventilating) and had a funny feeling in her tummy. Her husband Greg agreed to rearrange his day to drive her to work.

At the church prayer meeting that evening Helen prevailed upon Amanda to drive her to work for the rest of the week. But Helen became very anxious and had a panic attack the following evening when she would normally have done her usual weekly shop at Asda. She didn't go, and instead spent a stressful evening doing her shopping online. Over the following weeks Helen was edgy much of the time, with fluctuating muscular tension, headaches, hyperventilation and tingling. At times she became sad and tearful. She stopped going to the Sunday services because they were so busy and crowded. She could only cope with the midweek meeting if Greg or Amanda were available to take her there and home again. She didn't return to Asda or to any shops. She would only ever go out with Greg or Amanda. When she had a panic attack on a busy day at the office, she stopped going to work too.

Greg then asked their GP to visit and he referred her to a psychiatrist who diagnosed agoraphobia and arranged for a psychologist to work with her on a programme of graded exposure (a behavioural treatment) and anxiety management. Amanda and others at church visited and spent time reading and praying with her. They encouraged her to set a schedule at home, with regular meals and exercise, and to practise good sleep hygiene. Her anxiety settled slowly, and the panic attacks stopped. Helen was eventually able to resume work and full involvement at church, using the bus and shops as normal.

Agoraphobia involves fear of overcrowded places. Commonly, sufferers have long-standing generalized anxiety (which, unusually, Helen didn't), and the anxiety escalates into episodes of fear and panic when they feel trapped. Depressive symptoms and background stress can increase the vulnerability to such episodes. As with Helen, a consistent psychological approach is needed and medication is best avoided.

Key chapter points

- Psychosomatic illnesses overlap with what are often regarded as physical illnesses.

- There are no clear boundaries with these illnesses or with normality.
- A stepped-care approach utilizing straightforward measures can be implemented by church leaders to help people with mental illnesses (both psychosomatic illnesses and the severe mental illnesses of the next chapter).
- People with more severe psychosomatic illnesses require medical and sometimes specialist psychiatric help.

9. SEVERE MENTAL ILLNESSES: SCHIZOPHRENIA, DEMENTIA, BIPOLAR DISORDER AND DEPRESSION

Three anglers met up after their holidays. 'I caught a huge trout,' said one. 'Oh, but I caught a gigantic one,' responded his friend. The third jumped in with 'Well, mine was enormous', believing he had surely triumphed with the biggest catch of them all. Without a tape measure or weighing scales to determine the size of each fish, who could tell? So what justifies calling the illnesses in this chapter 'severe'?

Severe mental illnesses (SMI)[1] is a well-worn term in psychiatry services. It has currency. It is understood to refer to the kinds of illnesses that form the 'bread and butter' of specialist psychiatry practice in the NHS. People with these need assessment in, and most of their care provided by, such services and they often spend long periods as inpatients on psychiatric wards.

On the other hand, the psychosomatic illnesses of the previous chapter are usually dealt with predominantly in primary care, or with only brief contact with psychiatry services. Only rarely do the sufferers become inpatients. However, some people with psychosomatic illnesses are severely ill. The SMI term does not imply that psychosomatic illnesses are never severe, let alone trivial.

SMI encompasses the subcategories of mental illness that we will consider in this chapter: schizophrenia, dementia, bipolar disorder and depression. Although the terminology has varied, these are illnesses that have appeared throughout history. They also have a solid biological basis with identifiable brain changes. And they tend to do better with physical treatments (drugs and ECT) than psychological ones.

But psychological factors can play an important role in episodes of SMI, and CBT can be an important component in their treatment. Such CBT requires expertise. While elements of CBT can be usefully employed by a wide range of therapists for psychosomatic illnesses, in SMI specialists are needed because of the complexity and severity of these illnesses.

The principal difference in symptoms between SMI and psychosomatic illnesses is that people with SMI have cognitive and psychotic symptoms. All have deficits in cognition characterized by problems with memory and reasoning and so on. These cognitive symptoms are most obvious for people with dementia, but are there in milder form in those with other SMI. Psychotic symptoms, such as hallucinations and delusions, are most associated with schizophrenia, but are common in severer forms of bipolar and depressive illnesses, and also in dementia.

We conclude this book with short case examples and summaries of SMI, with links to websites where further detailed, accurate and reliable information can be found.

Schizophrenia

Can you imagine believing that those people standing over there can read your mind? Can you imagine being convinced that all your intimate thoughts are broadcast to everyone around you? Can you imagine not being sure whether what you think you hear is people talking about you, or whether it is just your own thoughts? Can you imagine the experience of your own body being manipulated by alien forces?

This is difficult, I know. A lot of the experiences of people with schizophrenia are non-understandable. I can understand someone feeling sad with depression, or having memory problems with dementia, because I get sad or forget things sometimes too. But I've never had those sorts of experiences.

These are the kinds of distressing experiences people with schizophrenia have when they are acutely ill. The essence of schizophrenia is the loss of that distinction between me and my private inner world and the rest of creation beyond myself. Schizophrenia is not 'split personality'. Rather, something like the opposite: a removal of that separation we take for granted between ourselves and everyone else. The illness breaks down these 'ego boundaries', leading to all sorts of weird and unpleasant experiences.

While auditory hallucinations ('hearing voices') may occur in several illnesses such as depression and dementia, they are characteristic of schizophrenia. When teaching, I say to students, 'Can you hear me OK?' And when they reply (hopefully!), 'Yes', I say this is how people hear voices when they have schizophrenia. Their auditory hallucinations are as real as this to them. It is just that there is no-one out there talking.

Mick used to talk about the 'mythomach', which was some kind of machine he believed aliens had installed in Northumberland. This 'mythomach' hoovered up all his thoughts, which were then stored to be used against him if he didn't comply. It also put their instructions into his mind. He was vague as to what exactly they wanted him to do, but nevertheless absolutely convinced and consequently terrified. Understandably, he had related persecutory beliefs that these aliens were after him. We would be paranoid too, wouldn't we, if we had such experiences? It must be very difficult to trust, and engage openly with, other people if you are unsure how much they can read or interfere with your thoughts.

Mick's paranoid beliefs were delusional, and typical of the kind of bizarre delusions people with schizophrenia often have as they struggle to make sense of their experiences. A delusion is a 'false, unshakeable belief, which is out of keeping with the patient's social and cultural background'.[2] This standard definition includes a part about a delusion not being culturally determined. This is to guard against labelling as mentally ill those whose views you disagree with.

Richard Dawkins, by entitling his book *The God Delusion*, has very unhelpfully propagated the erroneous view that a delusion is simply a belief I disagree with. Since far more people have always been theists than atheists, I might with more evidence and reason claim that it is Dawkins who is deluded (2 Thessalonians 2:11). I doubt Dawkins really meant to use 'delusion' in its proper psychiatric sense. Rather, he used it because calling your opponents deluded is a cheap way of belittling them at the expense of the genuinely mentally ill. But by using it wrongly, he has further muddied the waters in a tricky area.[3]

Schizophrenia can also disorder our thinking and language. As with Mick's 'mythomach', this may take the form of inventing new words and terms (neologisms). But it also damages the ability to form sentences properly, and so to think and speak coherently. This 'thought disorder' is another aspect of the illness that can make relationships with people with schizophrenia difficult when they have such symptoms. Our image-ness includes our ability to communicate, because God is a communicating God. This is crucial to forming and nurturing relationships with other people and with God.

Positive and negative symptoms

So far we have considered what we call positive symptoms of schizophrenia: hallucinations, delusions and thought disorder, symptoms that add to experience. Negative symptoms subtract from experience. They reduce the richness of life. People experience a flattening of their emotions, a blunting of the normal variation in their feelings, so that life feels rather grey. They speak less than others do and show a decreased range of spontaneous bodily movement. The drive to do things is also affected, so they become apathetic. They lose their 'get-up-and-go'. This can annoy others who think they are being lazy. Sometimes these features are a consequence of medication. But they are also a part of the illness itself.

Dementia praecox

Dementia praecox means premature dementia. It is what schizophrenia used to be called. Although it sounds peculiar, it helps us remember that part of schizophrenia is having cognitive problems, similar to those in mild dementia.

People with schizophrenia can also have marked changes in mood, usually sadness, but also many of the features of anxiety. Obsessional thoughts and rituals are frequent and well recognized as part of the illness. In fact, schizophrenia can cause any of the psychiatric symptoms characteristic of other mental illnesses.

Who gets schizophrenia?

Anyone can get schizophrenia. It is strongly genetic and so 'runs in families', but it occurs in people of all intellects and social classes all over the world and has done down the ages. About 1% of us will get it in our lives, and at any time about 0.5% are afflicted by it. It usually begins in early adult life. But it can begin at any age, and so I see people every year with schizophrenia commencing in old age.

Treatment of schizophrenia

Someone who is ill with acute schizophrenia, suffering a lot of delusions and hallucinations, needs urgent treatment with antipsychotic drugs. And this usually needs to take place in hospital. These drugs were developed over half a century ago and have proven of immense overall benefit to people with schizophrenia.[4] There are many individual drugs available. Pharmaceutical companies like to claim that newer drugs are better than the older ones. Unfortunately this is not the case. They have similar benefits, but different side effects. This means some people might prefer different drugs, and it is good to have a range of options.[5]

The most important side effects[6] include constipation, dry mouth and blurred vision; weight gain and changes in blood sugar and lipids; drops in blood pressure and dizziness; and stiffness, slowness and tremor. These can be troublesome, and it is understandable why some people are reluctant to take such drugs, especially once they have recovered and feel well.

Most sufferers benefit from antipsychotics, although it may take weeks and sometimes months before someone is well enough to leave hospital. After that there is often a longer period of further recovery.

Non-drug treatments

The onset of schizophrenia in early adulthood often leads to great difficulties because it interferes with education and training, which can have lasting effects on life outcomes. Thus, along with antipsychotic medication, social and psychological interventions are crucial. Social and vocational skills training themselves can be important in helping people overcome the impact of the illness.

Learning or relearning how to function in the workplace and elsewhere is important because, as we know, work is a key component of our service of God and as his image-bearers, for it helps us to function maturely as human beings. Recovering from an acute episode is slow and can take many months. Here, support from carers and family and friends is crucial because such relationships are another key aspect of our image-ness. Here also, the kind of counsel we discussed in chapter 7 from Christian leaders is important, as is social support from the church. And we need to remember also to care for the carers. Having a family member with schizophrenia (or any SMI) is hard and extremely draining.

Psychoeducation to help patients in understanding their illness and to encourage engagement with services is a core part of management. This also includes relapse recognition, helping the patient identify any early signs that a new episode might be developing. Formal family therapies are often employed because of the importance of families in care. But, at the least, involvement of key family and friends in some of the psychoeducation should occur, helping them to better understand the illness and support the patient.

CBT is increasingly used in schizophrenia as a supplement alongside medication.[7] Therapists work to help patients cope better with their stressors by identifying them and working out how to deal with them. CBT for schizophrenia focuses on the positive symptoms. This may sound surprising. How do you reason about what is un-understandable?

Well, you try to normalize the experience. For example, we all seek evidence to support what we believe, tending to ignore what might contradict us. This 'confirmation bias' is an approach these patients often use to support delusions too. So in CBT, patients are encouraged to think of alternative explanations for their experiences and evidence that contradicts their delusions. Sometimes we may make suggestions. But it is better if patients generate their own contradictory evidence. So with Mick, we would encourage him to think about why, if the aliens could invent such a powerful machine as the mythomach, they hadn't managed to 'get him' already?

CBT for schizophrenia requires skilled and experienced therapists and is frequently not available. But where available, it can be a helpful addition to medication and the other non-drug aspects of treatment.

Long-term outcomes

The longer-term outcome for people with schizophrenia is very variable. Some people, perhaps a fifth, get one episode only. Most experience further episodes, with some never fully recovering from their first one. Once patients have had two acute episodes, they are very likely to get more in future. This is important because it helps when discussing how long people should continue to take antipsychotic drugs.

Evidence supports the lifelong use of antipsychotics in such people. This is hard. Taking medication long term is not easy for any of us, and these drugs can cause unpleasant side effects. But even after many years, if drug treatment is stopped, relapse is likely. I've had several people who have stopped medication after decades of treatment. All have suffered another acute episode.

An experience of schizophrenia

I was upset when my church prayed about my heart
disease. I had been rushed to hospital with chest pain,
diagnosed as having a heart attack and treated with drugs.
Subsequent tests showed I had severe 'coronary heart
disease', and I had urgent insertions of coronary stents
that led to me being much better. But I cried when I learned
how the people at church had prayed for me because I
remembered how different it was over twenty years before
when I became acutely ill with schizophrenia. There had
been no church prayers then when I spent months severely
ill in hospital, and I and my parents had been unable even
to raise the issue and speak about it openly because of the
well-meaning ignorance we came up against whenever
we mentioned the subject. People didn't take the time
to find out what was going on and jumped to the conclusion
that I should grow up and snap out of it. They even tried
to persuade me to reject any drug treatment. You can
imagine how helpful this was to a young woman who
truly believed that the world was plotting together to
poison her.

What were the worst things for me back then? Standing
around the corner of the church car park unable to enter
the building for fear of who would be reading my thoughts
today, and hearing what their thoughts were saying about
me. The voices telling me to jump out of a fifth-floor
window at work. The fears about the plot to poison me and
take away my freedom. Shutting myself in my room every
time anyone came to our house. These still upset me now
when I remember them.

Also upsetting was hearing my parents tell the psychiatrist
how distressing it was for them helplessly to observe the
concentration, thinking, motivation and 'will to live'

disappearing from their lively and intelligent girl. They were upset when they saw my changed behaviour being misunderstood by well-meaning friends and family members who thought they knew best and were trying to help. They saw how the medication seemed to take away my personality and make me like 'a dead person inside a living body'.

What were the things that got us through? The private prayers of God's people: even though they didn't understand and couldn't talk publicly, I learned that on their own and at home many had lovingly prayed for me. I know it made all the difference. The word of God says, 'The words of the LORD are pure words, like silver refined in a furnace on the ground, purified seven times' (Psalm 12:6 ESV). There is no situation where God's word will not help us, and I found it spoke powerfully, straight at my need. The medication – praise to our ever-gracious God, in among all the debilitating side effects – did do what it was supposed to do and made me better.

I think my life has been different with my schizophrenia from what it would have been otherwise. I couldn't do as well in my career, but I am grateful to God for my parents and my husband. Most importantly of all, I will never again think of this world as a permanent residence, but I have my eyes fixed on the one that is to come.

Further reading

There is, of course, a vast amount of information available about schizophrenia on the internet, some the type of academic literature I read and much the kind that no-one should read. There are also websites with helpful information aimed at non-specialists, and if you wish to read further you might consider the following:

The charity Mind has a helpful booklet that can be downloaded, and videos of people describing their experience of schizophrenia:
http://www.mind.org.uk/information-support/
types-of-mental-health-problems/schizophrenia/
?gclid=CKOtzK6B384CFQWfGwod_toIBg#.V8AvIYdTGEV

The UK Royal College of Psychiatrists has a much more detailed summary of all aspects of schizophrenia, written at the general level:
http://www.rcpsych.ac.uk/healthadvice/problemsdisorders/
schizophrenia.aspx

Dementia

Dementia is not just memory problems. Dementia is not the same as Alzheimer's disease. I repeat these two statements like a record stuck in its groove (for those who remember vinyl records). Memory problems (amnesia) are the most well-known feature of dementia. Characteristically, dementia begins with loss of the ability to learn new information. Everyday meetings, appointments and so on get forgotten and objects get lost in the house. Over time the amnesia extends further back. But initially people retain a good memory for events earlier in their lives.

But dementia also causes problems with other aspects of cognition. People lose the ability to handle language. They often struggle to follow what you are saying because they can't process the words properly. They find it increasingly hard to concentrate and they lose track of what they are saying or doing. Their ability to recognize other people and objects gets damaged too. So they can get muddled about what a telephone is, or who this visitor is when their daughter pops in.

These various cognitive problems lead to difficulties in their everyday lives, what are called 'activities of daily living'. Initially, people can't carry out more complex activities, such as paying bills, driving a car or using appliances such as the washing machine or satellite TV. Later they struggle with easier tasks such as cooking. Finally, they need help with basic activities such as dressing and washing.

The memory isn't the problem

Families of people with dementia usually say they can cope with the memory problems. Using prompts and lists they can manage the forgetfulness. And patients are rarely worried. After all, you need to be able to remember in order to know you can't remember! This is what I tell people when I visit and they don't believe they have any problems (which is usually the case).

The other cognitive problems can be more difficult. When someone can't use language properly, they get understandably frustrated. And so do family and friends when communication is impaired. Again, when a mother fails to recognize her daughter and tells her to get out of the house, it is very distressing.

Difficulties in carrying out everyday activities, while annoying to people with dementia and their families, can be managed most of the time with extra support from family, neighbours or formal carers from social services.

Behavioural disturbance

But the big problems are behavioural.[8] Almost all people with dementia get several of these. They often experience distressing psychotic symptoms, as we saw with Malcolm's visual hallucinations in chapter 7. Depression, usually short-lived and mild, occurs in most people at some point, but occasionally some get a more severe depression which needs medication.

Apathy afflicts almost everyone. This involves a profound loss of drive, so people sit around doing nothing and need to be strongly encouraged to engage in activities they once enjoyed. Apathy is not depression. Those who experience apathy feel fine. They will smile and chat to you. But they won't do things without others pushing them, which is very frustrating.

Disinhibited behaviour is also common and can be highly embarrassing for friends and family. Agitation occurs in many people. They become restless and pace around appearing distressed. Wandering due to agitation is a common reason why people with dementia need to go to live in twenty-four-hour residential care.

Sleep disturbance can be extremely distressing for a spouse. The person with dementia typically wakes in the middle of the night, gets dressed and tries to go out. When this happens night after night, the patient and the spouse become exhausted. All these behavioural symptoms usually cause distress to the patients and almost always cause distress to family and carers who are more aware of them.

Dementia is more than Alzheimer's disease

Alzheimer's disease is a subset of dementia. In older people there are three major causes that account for the vast majority (more than 95%) of dementia: Alzheimer's disease (50–60%), Lewy body dementia (10–15%, consisting of two types: dementia with Lewy bodies and Parkinson's disease dementia) and vascular dementia (10–15%). I can do maths. These figures don't add up to more than 95% and the reason is because many people, especially the old-old (over eighty years), have more than one of these. In younger people fronto-temporal dementia is an important additional cause of dementia. And there are many other rarer causes, such as Huntington's disease and HIV disease.

Treatment of dementia

After someone has been diagnosed, he or she should receive information and advice. An assessment by a specialist social worker should be offered to discuss key aspects of future care. This includes a financial assessment, discussion on who will look after finances and property, advice on what home and day-care services are available, and information about carer support. Carer support is vital for the many family carers who bear the heavy burden of supporting a loved one with dementia.

For people with Alzheimer's disease there are two types of drug available that can improve the cognitive problems: the cholinesterase inhibitors (donepezil, galantamine, rivastigmine) and memantine. Each is widely prescribed and helpful for most sufferers. They each can also improve some of the other distressing symptoms, such as agitation and hallucinations.

Most people take the cholinesterase inhibitors without any noticeable side effects. Some lose their appetite and occasionally feel sickly or have tummy discomfort or loose stools. Other side effects are rare. Memantine has even fewer side effects.

These drugs are also widely prescribed for treating Lewy body dementia, and are especially helpful for visual hallucinations, agitation and aggression. They are not effective, though, in vascular dementia or fronto-temporal dementia, and probably not in other rarer causes.

People with Lewy body dementia usually have problems with movement due to the condition causing features of Parkinson's disease (it is in fact the same brain disorder). So they can benefit from treatments used for Parkinson's disease.

All these treatments improve the symptoms without altering the progression of the diseases. Unfortunately, there are no treatments available that slow down or stop any of the diseases causing dementia.

Treating behavioural problems

Psychosis-driven agitation and aggression can be effectively treated with antipsychotic drugs. Low doses can produce immense benefits for patient and family. Historically, these drugs were overprescribed, being used for all sorts of mild behavioural problems. We now know they have significant risks. But frequently the distress due to the psychosis or agitation is so great that the benefits outweigh these risks. It is better to have a settled and contented patient and family with this small risk than months, and perhaps years, of misery.

Some people with depression in dementia have a depression that responds to antidepressants. But most do not. There are many understandable reasons why people with dementia feel depressed. They lack conversation and social engagement. They need pain treatment or laxatives for constipation.

Hypnotic drugs (sleeping tablets) are usually effective for sleep disturbance. These are the same type of drug as the 'minor tranquillizers' used to treat anxiety. They need careful use because of the risk of hangover sedation. This is when people remain a little sedated the next day, and may become more confused and more likely to fall and injure themselves.

Non-drug treatments

Most of the important care for people with dementia does not come from medication. In the early stages patients can be helped by engagement in social events, and formal treatment in health services with non-drug treatments like cognitive-stimulation therapy.

Later, non-drug approaches to help with behavioural problems can be effective and avoid the need for medication. These work in most people with milder problems, with the above drug treatments reserved for more severe disturbance. Sometimes the behaviour cannot be managed at home, so admission to a care home or a specialist hospital unit is needed.

Not everyone with dementia goes to a care home. But many people reach a point at which they can no longer be looked after at home. They may move to a supported care facility, where carers are available when needed, or to a twenty-four-hour nursing home, where carers are present all the time.

How can the church help people with dementia?

Every church with some older members will have people with dementia. It affects a tenth of those over seventy and a fifth of those over eighty. Of course this means, contrary to some perceptions, that most older people don't have dementia. In some cases it might not be recognized, and perhaps when a diagnosis is made it is not widely known in the church.

Individuals with dementia should inform the church leaders of their diagnosis, as well as those they know best. Or if people in a church suspect it, they can sensitively raise this in private and encourage them to have a medical assessment. In the earlier stages people will become repetitive in conversation. Impaired concentration and amnesia can lead them to lose track of a conversation. Language impairment, affecting their comprehension and their ability to express themselves, is frequently present too. Speaking a little more slowly (while avoiding appearing patronizing) and using short sentences can help.

As the dementia progresses, this difficulty in understanding can lead to sufferers talking aloud inappropriately. They may ask for help and become restless and agitated. At this point it is likely that continued attendance at church services is no longer appropriate. The person with dementia can't comprehend in order to benefit or contribute and is instead confused and distressed.

To meet the needs of such older people, a church may run luncheon clubs or other special daytime meetings. This maintains their involvement with the Lord's people and connection with their church. Churches may also run services within nursing homes to help Christians who cannot get out.

People in churches can help in practical ways by giving lifts, taking people out for trips to relieve the burden on the spouse, and simply by visiting. Regular visits from members can help retain contact with their church. Such visits and services will need to be brief, clear and simple in order to maximize the opportunity for those with more advanced dementia to participate.

People with severe dementia, who can't speak clearly and struggle to comprehend our speech, remain aware of our body language. Thus they can be rightly upset and angered by individuals who talk about them in front of them. While they may not fully understand all that is being said, they do perceive a bad attitude and a lack of respect.

Positively, though, this means we can communicate our love and care for them by maintaining eye contact, smiling and talking kindly to them. A little touch, a gentle kiss and a short prayer will still speak effectively to them of a family's care and of our love for them in Christ. While it may be difficult to know how much of what we say is understood by people with severe dementia, there are frequently indications that more is grasped than we might think.

Christians enjoy a direct personal communion with God that transcends understanding. Our experience of the Lord does not have to involve conscious, intelligent comprehension. When the unborn John the Baptist encountered Mary carrying Jesus in her womb, he was moved by the Spirit to leap for joy in recognition of his Saviour (Luke 1:41, 44). At this foetal stage of development he could not use language or reason. But nonetheless, God the Holy Spirit caused him to express himself in such devotion to Jesus. Thus, even when people with dementia have lost their language skills and can no longer think or communicate in such ways, they are still able to receive real blessings from the Lord.

Well-learned, long-standing habits are retained much better. Thus, if a Christian has for years been regular and diligent in prayer and daily made time to read and reflect on the Scriptures, then these good habits will remain for a long time. If believers have ingrained their attendance at church services on the Lord's Day, then they will continue to want to do this.

A related point is that a regular ordered church service structure makes it a lot easier for people with dementia to settle and engage with the worship. Familiarity with the regular rhythm of worship is retained in early dementia. Conversely, if a church changes its pattern of worship, especially if it does so frequently, then they will find it much harder to be settled in these services.

What do we do when those with dementia become agitated during a service? Prevention is better than cure. If they have no family at church, then a church leader or friend can sit beside them to reassure and comfort them and assist them in opening a Bible or hymnbook or receiving Communion. If this fails, then, sadly, it is likely that they need to cease attendance.

How do we respond to bad behaviour? We saw in chapter 6 that in the milder and earlier stages people retain their mental capacity and know the difference between right and wrong. Such knowledge is ingrained and not lost until someone is severely impaired. Thus, for example, it may be appropriate to rebuke someone who sins by becoming angry or aggressive if we would do the same to someone without dementia.

However, even when sufferers retain their mental capacity and know their behaviour was sinful, we remember they are ill. So we respond with compassion. A seventy-two-year-old with dementia who hits out at his wife in anger needs handling very differently from a forty-year-old wife-beater. His behaviour is influenced by misinterpretations of her words due to his language problems and other aspects of dementia. She can rightly rebuke him for such an outburst, but does so knowing 'he is not himself'. She does so with sympathy and gentleness.

An experience of dementia

Dad used to live down the road from us after Mum died. I'd always be popping in after work on my way home. As a district nurse, I knew a lot of folk who had struggled with the role reversals that come when a close relative develops dementia and needs caring for. Well, when Dad started with dementia, I was used to all the things that could go along with that: the caring for and protecting, the urging and coaxing, the helping with bathing and personal care, and the difficulties in getting changes of clothes on or tablets swallowed.

But what I wasn't prepared for was the effect on our father–daughter relationship. Yes, I felt as a carer more like the parent than the child, the one who was to protect rather than the one who is protected and looked after. But it's natural to want to care for your loved one, and so that role reversal just somehow felt natural too.

When Dad needed more care, he moved in with us. It was fine at first, but after a while he started acting strangely. He would be irritable at times and at others he'd be putting his arm around folk like the plumber and chattering on to strangers as if they were his long-lost brothers. I thought to myself, 'He's becoming a bit over-friendly', but then he started turning his attention on me. His usual goodnight peck on the cheek became less appropriate attempts at affection. It was bewildering and devastating. I thought I'd just been mistaken, but no, the behaviour continued, and where I'd always loved and respected my dad even in his dementia state, I was now scared to be alone in the room with him. I couldn't say anything to anyone about it. I didn't despise him or anything. I just didn't want him to treat me as if I was his wife. I was his daughter. It was awful having our father–daughter relationship wrenched apart. I knew at this point that I couldn't manage to care for him myself any more. I felt a real failure, guilty for distancing myself from him in a seemingly unloving way. Arranging his move into a care home felt like the height of cruelty on my part, a betrayal. But he developed a pneumonia following a fall, and the move never happened as he died in hospital.

However, what has stayed with me is this lasting memory of my attempted betrayal and his misdirected attentions to me. Perhaps he was thinking I was my mum when she was my age. It is sad, and so I try to dwell on good times and what was precious in our relationship in better times.

Further reading

Again, the internet is awash with websites about dementia. Two major UK dementia charities supply accurate and readable factsheets and other information:

http://alzheimers.org.uk/factsheets
http://www.alzheimersresearchuk.org/
dementia-information/

Bipolar disorder

He didn't have time to talk with me. They were busy filming the next episode of *Pirates of the Caribbean* down at the quayside in Newcastle. Johnny Depp, Orlando Bloom, Keira Knightley, they were all there. But the leading figure in this new movie was the man in front of me, Kevin Smith. His would be the name above the title.

I explained that while not a movie expert, I'd never heard of Kevin Smith. He told me I was stupid. He was a new kind of Hollywood megastar. The anonymous kind. My mind boggled. I moved on and said I'd been at the quayside a few times in recent weeks and had never noticed any film-making. With ill-concealed contempt, he explained, 'You know the Harry Potter films? He has an invisibility cloak. Well, we have a very big one, so we can film without anyone seeing.'

Kevin had grandiose delusions and had been admitted under the Mental Health Act with acute mania. He hadn't slept for several days but was still brimming with energy. And with sexual vitality. The cause of his admission had been his persistent attempts to seduce women in the Newcastle clubs. Believing he was such a megastar, he was annoyed they wouldn't fall into bed with him. Their boyfriends weren't too pleased either.

He had also spent large sums of money funding his extravagant film-star lifestyle in different hotels around England, as he had rushed from one city to another. Sums which Kevin Smith, the joiner, would find hard to pay. His mood was elated (very high) and his speech fast and at times difficult to follow.

Manic depression no more

Bipolar disorder used to be called 'manic depression',[9] and sometimes that phrase is still used. It is so named because people swing between two mood poles: mania and depression. The illness typically consists of a series of episodes, usually more manic episodes when people are younger and more depression as they get older.

The manic pole experienced by Kevin is unique to this mental illness, and Kevin had all the symptoms of acute mania. Usually, and especially when on treatment, the manic phases are a little milder. But most of the time people with bipolar suffer from depression rather than mania. These episodes are essentially the same as those in depressive illness, which we will look at below.

How common is bipolar disorder?

Bipolar disorder affects about 2% of the world's population and, like schizophrenia, it is 'no respecter of persons'.[10] That is, it afflicts anyone; it does not discriminate. It affects men and women equally and begins early in life, in late teens and twenties in most.

Hospital treatment is usually required for manic episodes and for more severe depressive episodes. Recovery from the more severe features – delusions and not sleeping – takes a few weeks, but it usually takes several months for people to return to normal. Hence they can be unwell for a long period after they have returned home from hospital.

People with bipolar disorder typically get multiple episodes over their lifetime and can end up with a significant proportion of their time unwell with mania or depression. This is a huge burden for them and their families.

Helping people with bipolar disorder

The consequences of acute mania can be devastating. Think about the after-effects for Kevin when he got well. He had huge debts. His employment was in jeopardy because he had neglected his customers when he was ill, and his marriage was strained by his attempted infidelity. Thus again, helping people with this illness requires much more than medication, and church members are well placed to provide support and practical help.

Treatment of bipolar disorder[11]

Treatment for a manic episode involves medication with antipsychotics, or other drugs such as lithium. When mania is most severe, the drugs frequently need to be given initially by injection until someone is settled enough to take tablets. The drug treatment of the depression is complex because of the risk of antidepressants provoking an episode of mania, and so combination treatments are usually used.

Once patients have settled on medication, then psychoeducation has a key role, especially following a first episode, to help them understand their illness. Aims include reducing the risk of future episodes by avoiding triggers, and encouraging compliance with medication. CBT can add value at this stage too and reduce the long-term risk of future episodes.[12]

In bipolar disorder, CBT is usually given when people have largely recovered from the manic or depressive episode. It is used along with drug treatment, and overall the combination tends to produce better outcomes. People recovering from mania tend to have unrealistically positive thinking patterns, for example thinking they are invincible and so taking on all comers in fights in nightclubs. Or like Kevin, thinking all women must find them sexually attractive and irresistible. CBT can help to encourage a more realistic self-perception.

The risk of future episodes in someone with bipolar disorder is very high, so long-term drug treatment with lithium, valproate or antipsychotics should be encouraged even after one episode. Since first episodes often occur when people are young, this can be very difficult, as sufferers are understandably reluctant to take medication for the foreseeable future. Good engagement and psychoeducation are needed to help individuals weigh up the risks and benefits for themselves.

Lithium needs to be carefully monitored with regular blood checks, because if the level gets too high, it can cause serious problems with slurred speech, double vision, shaking arms and unsteady walking. At normal treatment levels it can cause a mild tremor, tummy problems, thirstiness and a frequent need to go to the toilet.

Valproate is quite sedative and may cause tremor, unsteadiness and tummy problems (sickness, pain and either diarrhoea or constipation). Importantly, both lithium and valproate can cause damage to the unborn child and so should be avoided if possible during pregnancy.

The impact of mental illness (bipolar disorder) on a family
When mental illness hits a person's life, it is like a stone hitting a lake. The impact of that stone affects those around in ever-expanding concentric circles. This impact is often felt most strongly by the family.

Unlike a broken bone, this type of illness is not easily fixed by plaster or surgery. Its impact on a family lasts for years, not weeks, sometimes a lifetime. It remains hidden, sometimes unspoken. For some, there is guilt attached. A suggestion by a nurse that the family may have been repressive causes them to wonder, what if . . . ?

Nor is this impact constant or easily quantifiable. To live with someone with bipolar in particular is like sharing a rollercoaster ride. There are moments of elation as 'normality' seems close, or despair as mania or depression reappear. Underneath all these emotions lurks fear: a fear of what that loved ones might do, either to themselves or to those closest to them; a fear of what the future may hold; a fear of the impact of their behaviour on the children in the family.

Yet not every impact is negative. To go to places you'd never imagined, to see a fellow human so open and raw, can draw from the heart a tenderness that hurts. It reminds us of our own fragility and strips away the trappings of society. We see someone made in the image of God, and it calls forth a godlike response: compassion.

Further reading

Again, for more information on bipolar disorder, the UK charity Mind and the Royal College of Psychiatrists have information freely available from their websites at these addresses:
http://www.mind.org.uk/information-support/
types-of-mental-health-problems/bipolar-disorder/
about-bipolar-disorder/?o=1142#.V-kIEPArK70
http://www.rcpsych.ac.uk/healthadvice/problemsdisorders/
bipolardisorder.aspx

Depression

'When I use a word,' Humpty Dumpty said, in rather a scornful tone, 'it means just what I choose it to mean – neither more nor less.' 'The question is,' said Alice, 'whether you can make words mean so many different things.'[13] Nowadays depression is a Humpty Dumpty word, one that people use to mean many different things.

Is it a bird? Is it a plane?

At a recent meeting a colleague likened our problem with depression to that of saying that everything that flies is a bird. Everyone with depression feels sad, but beyond that they are very different, as different as a bat or a mayfly is from a robin.

Unhappiness and stress due to the vicissitudes of life have been medicalized as 'depression'. It has become a twenty-first-century catch-all diagnosis – the common cold of mental illness. The diagnosis rates for depression have soared: 40% of people in nursing homes in the UK are on antidepressants, and 4.9% of all adults in the UK and 10% in the USA are taking antidepressants, making these the most commonly prescribed of all drugs.[14]

Yet some doctors claim we are still under-prescribing because there are studies telling us 20% of adults have 'depression' that needs treatment. This is not good. If you don't have an illness, then any drug treatment for it only gives you the side effects. You can't get the benefit, just the harms.

How we arrived at this position is fascinating (to some of us anyway), and medical historian Edward Shorter traces the expansion of depression to cover any kind of sadness in his book *How Everyone Became Depressed*.[15] Below we have four different examples of depression, which illustrate something of this variety.

Burnout

Kylie had been under huge pressure at work as a junior doctor. The repeated moves to training posts in new hospitals where she had to learn new systems and meet new people were themselves draining. The jobs were disappointing. They did not bring her the kind of pleasure she had hoped to experience as a doctor. Her sleep pattern was disrupted by the shift patterns, and she was trying to squeeze in study for her postgraduate exams while maintaining involvement in her church.

She felt miserable, exhausted, and often when back on her own at her flat she cried. Her mother told her she was depressed and should see her GP. She dutifully did so. Her friend Lucy, who was training in psychiatry, disagreed. Lucy thought Kylie was exhausted from overwork and needed a good break. Kylie's GP prescribed her fluoxetine and offered her a sick note. She decided she needed the break Lucy had suggested and enjoyed a restful week away from work. She felt much better and never took her fluoxetine.

Lucy was right. Kylie did not need to expose herself to the risks of unnecessary medication. The 'burnout' term more helpfully identifies Kylie's situation. Her predicament was perhaps similar to that of Elijah in 1 Kings 19. He was shattered following his highly stressful confrontation with the prophets of Baal and the physical effort of their slaughter. He then had to flee for his life over a large distance. And so the Lord ministered to his exhausted servant by giving him rest, food and drink. And encouragement and a human companion (Elisha).

Kylie needed further help, however. The way forward was for her to discuss her situation with some of her church leaders. Together they could work out a better weekly routine, endeavouring to get the 'stepped-care' basics right (see chapter 8). Getting help from a mature Christian friend to examine her life priorities would also be important. Perhaps Kylie would need to work part-time? Perhaps she should postpone her exams? She did need to make structural changes to her pattern of living to prevent future burnout.

Not so major depression

The diagnostic manual DSM has a term for depressive illness: 'major depressive disorder'. You might think that this is so-called because it contrasts with 'minor depressive disorder'. But it doesn't. There is no 'minor depression'. Instead, in the psychiatric equivalent of grade inflation in exams, all depression is major.

In routine clinical practice, few psychiatrists use the term 'major depression'. We just diagnose 'depression'. But this is used as an equivalent for major depression and covers the whole spectrum. Minor depression was abandoned for political reasons about forty years ago.[16] It had referred to the kind of psychosomatic illness we looked at in the previous chapter and which Liam has below. Its abandonment as a term is a shame because it would be helpful to flag up people who would benefit from psychological treatment rather than from antidepressants.

Minor depression

Liam's relationship with Denise had grown increasingly difficult. There had been problems for many months because of their working patterns. Each was trying to develop a career and juggle their shared responsibilities at home while raising their two young children.

But over the past couple of months Liam had been called in twice to report at work to his supervisor about his poor performance. This had never happened before. His customers had previously rated his performance highly. But not now.

His sleep pattern had become patchy and he avoided sexual contact with Denise. He was overeating and had put on weight. He felt miserable most of the time. Finally, he had to take time off work and his supervisor suggested he seek medical attention.

Taking time off work, Liam brought the situation to the attention of Tim, their pastor, who paid them a visit one evening. Tim had been aware of some strain in their marriage and had wondered about whether to get involved. Now they all recognized that some additional advice and support were needed. Tim encouraged them to think about their priorities and adjust their working lives so they had more time for each other and their children. And time to rest.

Liam's GP had done some psychiatry and did not reach for the prescription pad. Instead, he referred Liam for a course of CBT for his depression.[17] With the encouragement of Denise, he worked at this and made good progress. After six months he returned to his previous level of performance at work and became largely free of depressive symptoms.

Minor depressive illnesses like Liam's tend to come and go. They are often associated with the kinds of work and family-related stressors that Liam had. Where such factors are present, they need to be addressed, which in Liam's case was by pastoral intervention to help with marital stress. And by CBT to focus on the work-related pressures and on managing the depressive symptoms.

Moderate depressive illness

Ryan had been a pillar in his local church for years, quietly and faithfully serving as a deacon. He was respected and liked at work, where he had gradually climbed the ladder to his senior management position in human resources. He got flu one winter like everyone else, but unlike everyone else, he never recovered.

When the fever settled, his tiredness didn't go away. He became sadder and sadder. He found himself waking at 4 a.m. and feeling dead. All appetite for life seemed to have drained out of him, and he couldn't enjoy anything. Everything seemed greyed out. He hoped it would pass off, but instead he got worse.

When his wife couldn't persuade him to leave the house and he told her he wished he were dead, she called his GP. She visited that day and immediately started him on the antidepressant sertraline and referred him to local psychiatry services.

The psychiatrist visited later that week. He noted how Ryan avoided eye contact, sat hunched with little body movement and showed no responsiveness in conversation, only uttering a few quiet words in response to questions. Ryan admitted he felt so terrible he didn't want to live, but declared that as a Christian he had no suicidal thoughts.

The psychiatrist explained he had a moderately severe depressive illness, which should do well with the sertraline. He recommended that this be increased quickly as long as Ryan didn't get side effects, and explained what these might be. He arranged for a community nurse to visit, who monitored Ryan's progress and explained his illness and its implications (psychoeducation).

Ryan responded very well to the full standard dose of sertraline (150mg daily), returning to work and his regular lifestyle. But he was left with residual anxiety. He felt tense and edgy, with periods of more intense discomfort. His community nurse introduced CBT, with an emphasis on understanding and dealing with anxiety, and he recovered over the following months.

Antidepressants

Ryan's was the kind of more severe depressive illness which usually does well with medication. Contrary to oft-repeated claims, antidepressants are of proven benefit in moderate and severe depressive illnesses. But once you move back towards the blurred line with normal stressful experience, these benefits disappear.[18] For people like Liam with minor depression there is no clear benefit from such medication, and psychological approaches are more appropriate.

There are different categories of antidepressants. All are almost equally effective but have different side-effect profiles. The most commonly used are the selective serotonin reuptake inhibitors (SSRIs). Prozac is perhaps still the most famous. They can cause tummy problems (sickness, discomfort/pain, diarrhoea, vomiting), sexual problems, wakefulness and agitation. They may also cause bleeding in the tummy, and confusion, especially in older people.

The older antidepressants, for example amitriptyline, can lead to constipation, dry mouth and blurred vision; drops in blood pressure and dizziness; and sedation and weight gain. A commonly used but different antidepressant is mirtazapine, whose main side effects are sedation and weight gain.

More severe depressive illnesses like Ryan's recur. So antidepressants should be used for a long time after recovery from an illness episode. In older people this should be for the rest of life. In younger adults they should be continued for six to nine months after recovery from a first episode.

If there has been more than one episode, then medication should be used even longer. The duration of such treatment is a difficult decision that needs to be carefully worked out on a patient-by-patient basis. This involves discussion with the patient, who has to weigh up the potential impact of future episodes on his or her life against the tedium of long-term medication use and its associated adverse effects. Where CBT has been helpful, then it may also be used in the longer term, often as intermittent 'top-up' sessions with the therapist.

Psychotic depression

Penny had enjoyed a happy marriage to Frank and had coped when he died of cancer in his fifties. She had had to take up work again after this and settled well into life as a sales assistant. Then one July she began making mistakes, and customers complained that she was surly and rude. She felt exhausted all day long and 'like death warmed up' when she woke each morning.

Her children encouraged her to visit her GP who was very worried. She admitted she had virtually stopped eating because she had no interest in food any more. In fact, she didn't enjoy anything now. The GP weighed Penny and found she had lost a few kilogrammes. Her physical examination and blood tests were all normal. Her doctor made an urgent referral to psychiatry services and started her on the antidepressant citalopram.

When she was seen the following month, she had lost another three kilogrammes. Her daughter had driven up from Kent to be present and told the psychiatrist that Penny had been saying peculiar things about herself. She said she couldn't eat because she had no stomach, and even claimed that all her insides had dissolved.

Penny spoke little and hardly moved during the assessment.[19] She denied that she had any thoughts of killing herself, but said she would prefer to be dead. She simply lacked the courage to try to kill herself. She was asked about coming into hospital but declined. She agreed to double her dose of citalopram and to take an antipsychotic drug aripiprazole as well and to see a community nurse regularly.

When the nurse visited the next week, he found the aripiprazole had not been used. Penny complained about her neighbours. She blamed them for her condition, although it wasn't clear what she thought they had done. But she was clear that they were making nasty comments about her because she could hear them doing so. Since she lived in a detached house, these were recognized as auditory hallucinations, and she was again asked to come to hospital for treatment. She refused and had to be admitted under a section of the Mental Health Act.

In hospital she continued to hallucinate, refuse to eat and express delusional beliefs about her insides. She often lay down on the floor saying she was dead and refused to engage with anyone. Urgent ECT was arranged and after a few treatments she was markedly improved. She began eating and taking her medication. She started talking to people, albeit very little and with grim gloominess about her future and her health. After a few weeks of ECT, however, she was back to her normal self and taking all her medication.

Severe depression is often associated with psychotic symptoms that match the low mood of the patient. Penny's beliefs about her stomach and insides were typical of such (nihilistic) delusions. The kind of critical and persecutory hallucinations she experienced are also characteristic.

Such illnesses frequently advance quickly, and before any benefits from antidepressants become apparent, there can be rapid deterioration. This can lead to the antidepressants being blamed for making things worse. When people are psychotically depressed, there is no role for psychotherapy, although this can be used once people have recovered sufficiently to engage. Antipsychotics are of established benefit in such people. But when deterioration leads to the kind of weight loss and distressing psychosis that Penny experienced, then ECT is often needed and it is usually rapidly beneficial.

Following recovery, long-term treatment with antidepressants is needed. When antipsychotics have been helpful, then they too should be continued long term. Again, it can be difficult to decide how long to continue such therapy. When illness episodes have been as severe as Penny's, then patients often opt for lifelong treatment because of fear of such an episode recurring.

An experience of depression

I remember how we found Dad on the floor with the tablets around him. I will never forget this. I had been worried because he had become so gloomy and said he wasn't eating, so we visited and he seemed thin and quiet and very sad. I made him go to his GP, who put him on an antidepressant, but when we phoned, he just seemed worse. So we went again to take him to his bowling, which he had given up. That was when we found him. We used our key to get in when he wouldn't answer, and there he was, groaning on the floor.

We called the ambulance and went with him to hospital. He woke up while we waited but he just seemed so unwell. He told us we had abandoned him and that we wanted him to die. This was very upsetting. He said he had heard people talking to him telling him this, and so he should kill himself. The psychiatrist told us he had hallucinations and severe depression. He put him on a strong antidepressant and a drug to treat his hallucinations.

Dad continued not eating enough and often wouldn't drink. It was horrible seeing him like that. The weight just fell off him. He kept blaming us for putting him in hospital. He was sure what the voices had told him was true: we were trying to do bad things to him. Slowly, over weeks, he got better, but it seemed like months. When he was well he didn't remember anything about what had happened. I suppose this might be better because it is very difficult to think about it now – your own dad saying things like that.

He has been well for a long time now and still takes both his treatments. He has been told to keep taking them, but sometimes he says he won't – he doesn't see why he should because he hadn't really been that unwell. I dread him stopping them because it might happen all over again. It is odd that I am more worried about it than he is.

Further reading

If you want to read more about depression and its treatment, then the charity Mind has a helpful booklet which can be downloaded:

http://www.mind.org.uk/information-support/
types-of-mental-health-problems/depression/
about-depression/?o=9109#.V-j_o_ArK7o

And again, the Royal College of Psychiatrists has information on depression at:

http://www.rcpsych.ac.uk/healthadvice/problemsdisorders/
depression.aspx

Final thoughts

What makes a good doctor? It's an old conundrum. Is it someone with technical brilliance, immense knowledge, profound diagnostic skill and therapeutic excellence, but no people skills? A doctor exemplified by *Doc Martin* of the TV comedy? Or is it someone with compassion, who senses your pain, sympathizes with your problems, but whose medical competence leaves something to be desired? Of course, we want both expertise and compassion.

I believe Christian ministers and church leaders have both. Ministers contact me from time to time seeking my help. They have been trying to help people in their flock who have mental illness or distress. My strong conviction, repeated throughout this book, is that church leaders and mature Christian men and women are well placed to help. I've seen it work in practice. Indeed, this has been the major driver for my writing.

Patients want doctors who care. Good doctors cultivate warm relationships with patients. Even the experts (like me!) in the medical schools have embraced this truth. So these days all medical students are taught interpersonal skills. Indeed, a gripe among the professors and examiners nowadays is how much time the students spend doing 'the compassion bit'. Christians, and especially mature believers, should, and I believe do, excel in this. For we worship a God of love, whose compassion was clearly demonstrated in our Saviour during his ministry, characterized by helping and healing the sick and needy.

But we don't want only gushing sympathy. We want strength too. We need someone who not only connects with our suffering but who knows how to help us through it. There is a common fallacy that you can't help someone unless you've experienced the problem yourself. 'You don't know what I'm going through, doctor. Have you ever had schizophrenia?' No, thank God, I have not. But I've talked with many who have and have learned from them. Hebrews 4:15 encourages us that Jesus is able to be compassionate and help us. How? After all, he didn't experience all the same temptations as me. But he did go through temptations of the same kind (lust, pride, greed and so on). And crucially, he was successful. His victory over all of these is what fully equips him to help.

And church leaders have a wealth of relevant experience in helping people. This gives us transferable skills that prepare us for aiding the mentally ill. Like our Saviour, we don't experience each and every kind of problem. But we experience some and learn much more from helping others.

A little knowledge

They say a little knowledge is a dangerous thing. This book has given a little knowledge about mental illness and a framework for helping the mentally ill. But of course it will not equip anyone to replace the expertise of psychiatrists and other specialists in health services. It would be dangerous if anyone thought so, although I doubt anyone will. However, a little knowledge can also go a long way when it is wisely used to augment the experience and knowledge that Christian leaders already possess. Ministers can work together with people with milder mental illnesses and those in distress to tackle their problems effectively. And for people with severer illnesses, church leaders can work together with health services to complement their expertise.

Christian men and women also have important advantages over professionals in health services. We have a proper understanding of who we are, and we know that the mind has a major role in both illness and healing. We know everyone is made in God's image, whether mentally well or ill, and is therefore valuable and worthy of our efforts to help. We recognize that we were created for 'work', and so promote such activity for its benefits. And we appreciate the importance of personal relationships.

In our churches we have a tremendous resource for helping the mentally ill, through our church-family relationships. Our knowledge of one another and the bonds established in our fellowships provide a powerful resource that we can draw upon. Yes, sadly, too often there may have been stigma and ignorance leading to harm. But this need not be so. And I hope, as you finish this book, you will be someone who is not only free of negative perceptions of the mentally ill, but better informed and able to help and heal them. I pray you have indeed been instilled with the confidence to tackle mental illness together with patients, their families and health services.

Key chapter points

- Severe mental illnesses require specialist care, and inpatient care in hospital is frequently needed.
- Church leaders and churches can play an important supportive role during episodes of severe illness, as they do with physical illnesses.
- Between episodes we can be more actively engaged in care.
- Support for family members caring for people with severe mental illness is crucial.

GLOSSARY

CBT (Cognitive-behavioural therapy) is the most commonly used form of psychotherapy. In CBT there is a focus on both analysing the behaviours of patients and interpreting their thought processes accompanying these behaviours. Collaboratively the patient and therapist identify ways to deal with them.

Cognition refers to our intellectual faculties by which we concentrate, learn, remember and reason.

Delusions are false and fixed beliefs, which are not explained by someone's religious, cultural and social background. They are a major feature of psychotic illnesses.

Drugs We have a problem in English since the same word is used for both illegal ('street') drugs and medication. In this book 'drugs' used without qualification refers to medication used to treat illnesses and medical symptoms.

DSM (*The Diagnostic and Statistical Manual of Mental Disorders*; DSM, current version 5, published 2013) has often been called 'the bible of psychiatry'. It is the modern reference work for making psychiatric diagnoses.

ECT is electroconvulsive therapy, which is the most effective treatment for severe depression and beneficial in some other mental illnesses too.

Hallucinations are false perceptions. Most common are auditory hallucinations (hearing voices or sounds when no-one is speaking and nothing explains them) and visual hallucinations (seeing things which are not there). With delusions, they are the major type of psychotic symptom.

Hysteria is impossible to define. Today it tends to mean someone is highly emotional. But it was a widely used medical term to refer to people who experienced a kaleidoscopic range of physical and mental symptoms that were stress-related. In this book it is used in this medical way and is equivalent to 'psychosomatic illnesses'.

IPT (interpersonal psychotherapy) is a widely used psychotherapy, especially for depression. It places emphasis on the patient's relationships and problems related to these.

Neurosis is another historical term that defies definition. Neurosis refers to an exaggerated reaction to circumstances involving normal emotions such as anxiety or depression. It covers roughly the same group of psychosomatic symptoms as hysteria.

Psychoeducation refers to providing specific information about a mental illness, either written or at a consultation, to help people live better with their illness.

Psychosomatic is used to refer to humans as having both a physical body and a mind/spirit. These are united in one whole being. Thus all illnesses involve both body and mind/spirit. But sometimes this is especially prominent, and these are the 'psychosomatic illnesses' of this book.

Psychotic illnesses are those in which the sufferer is detached from objective reality. The hallmark symptoms of psychosis are delusions and hallucinations. Those suffering such illnesses often don't realize they are ill.

Side effects (adverse effects) are the unintended consequences of medical treatment.

SMI (severe mental illnesses) refers to a group of illnesses including schizophrenia, bipolar disorder, major depression and dementia.

SSRIs (selective serotonin reuptake inhibitors) are the most commonly prescribed type of antidepressant. The most well known is Prozac, the trade name for fluoxetine.

NOTES

Introduction: setting the scene

1. Andrew Scull, *Madness: A Very Short Introduction* (Oxford University Press, 2011), p. 3.
2. Timothy Rogers, *Trouble of Mind and the Disease of Melancholy* (Soli Deo Gloria, 2002), pp. 134–135.
3. Edward Shorter, *A History of Psychiatry: From the Era of the Asylum to the Age of Prozac* (John Wiley and Sons, 1997), pp. 1–2.
4. Ibid., p. 6.
5. Roger Carswell, *Where Is God in a Messed-up World?* (Inter-Varsity Press, 2006), pp. 109–110.
6. Ibid., p. 113.
7. I am grateful to Graham Heaps, retired pastor at Dewsbury Evangelical Church, for this observation.

1. It's not all in the mind

1. H. Merskey, *The Analysis of Hysteria: Understanding Conversion and Dissociation* (Royal College of Psychiatrists, 2006), pp. 11–12.
2. Jay E. Adams, *Competent to Counsel: Introduction to Nouthetic Counseling* (Zondervan, 1970), p. 28.
3. Jay E. Adams, *The Christian Counselor's Manual: The Practice of Nouthetic Counseling* (Baker, 1973), p. 11.

4. Heath Lambert, *The Biblical Counseling Movement after Adams* (Crossway, 2012). Lambert (p. 53) states that Adams initially allowed only two causes of 'problems in living': sin and organic illness. Later he added a third: 'There are in the Scriptures only three specified sources of personal problems in living: demonic activity (principally possession), personal sin and organic illness. These three are interrelated. All options are covered by these heads, leaving no room for a fourth: non-organic mental illness' (p. 9).

5. Gordon J. Wenham, *Genesis 1–15*, Word Biblical Commentary, vol. 1 (Word Books, 1987), p. 60.

6. Michael Horton, *The Christian Faith: A Systematic Theology for Pilgrims on the Way* (Zondervan, 2011), p. 379.

7. Ibid., p. 373.

8. See H. D. McDonald, 'Man, Doctrine of', in: W. A. Elwell (ed.), *Evangelical Dictionary of Theology* (Baker, 1984), p. 677.

9. Ibid.

10. Tom Burns, *Our Necessary Shadow: The Nature and Meaning of Psychiatry* (Allen Lane, 2013), p. 162.

11. Today these are often attributed to medication, but historical records demonstrate they are also due to the schizophrenia itself.

2. Rule and relationship

1. Roy Porter, *The Greatest Benefit to Mankind: A Medical History of Humanity from Antiquity to the Present* (HarperCollins, 1997), pp. 648–649.

2. See examples in Martin Gilbert, *The Second World War: A Complete History* (Phoenix Giant, 1989).

3. See Gordon J. Wenham, *Genesis 1–15*, Word Biblical Commentary, vol. 1 (Word Books, 1987), pp. 29–32; Peter J. Gentry and Stephen J. Wellum, *Kingdom through Covenant:*

A Biblical-Theological Understanding of the Covenants (Crossway, 2012), ch. 6.

4. Wenham, *Genesis 1–15*, p. 30.

5. Cited in Anthony A. Hoekema, *Created in God's Image* (Eerdmans, 1986), p. 66.

6. Michael Horton, *The Christian Faith: Systematic Theology for Pilgrims on the Way* (Zondervan, 2011), p. 387.

7. Ibid., pp. 70–71.

8. Outside the Genesis 'image contexts', the Hebrew word for 'image' is rarely used, and when it is used, it usually refers to physical objects which pictured and represented something, such as tumours (1 Samuel 6:5) or men (Ezekiel 16:17). Representativeness appears central to image: 'In the ancient East the setting up of the king's statue was the equivalent to the proclamation of his dominion over the sphere in which the statue was erected (cf. Daniel 3:1, 5f). When in the thirteenth century BC the Pharaoh Ramesses II had his image hewn out of the rock at the mouth of the *nahr el-kelb*, on the Mediterranean north of Beirut, the image meant that he was the ruler of this area.' See Hans Walter Wolff, *Anthropology of the Old Testament* (Fortress, 1974), pp. 160–161, cited in Gentry and Wellum, *Kingdom through Covenant*, ch. 6.

9. Hoekema, *Created in God's Image*, p. 76.

10. See Karl Popper and John C. Eccles, *The Self and Its Brain: An Argument for Interactionism* (Routledge, 1977), ch. P2.

3. What is mental illness?

1. *The Diagnostic and Statistical Manual of Mental Disorders* (DSM, current version 5, published 2013) has often been called 'the bible of psychiatry'. It is hugely influential, partly because its diagnostic categories are those used in the vast majority of psychiatric research studies and so shape clinical practice. Although in everyday work most psychiatrists only

apply the criteria loosely, we are unavoidably influenced by the DSM definition of, and approach to, mental disorders.

2. Allen Frances has brought together his published criticisms of *DSM-5* in his book, *Saving Normal* (HarperCollins, 2013).

3. Pyromania means repeatedly setting things on fire.

4. R. Moynihan, 'What Is Disease? And Why It's a Healthy Question', *BMJ* (2013), 346: f107.

5. Frances, *Saving Normal*. See also references to other critiques in this book.

6. *DSM-5* (p. 20) defines mental disorder as follows: 'A mental disorder is a *syndrome* characterised by *clinically significant disturbance* in an individual's cognition, emotion regulation, or behaviour that reflects a *dysfunction* in the psychological, biological or developmental processes underlying mental functioning. Mental disorders are usually associated with significant distress or disability in social, occupational, or other important activities. An *expectable or culturally approved response* to a common stressor or loss, such as the death of a loved one, is not a mental disorder. *Socially deviant behaviour* (e.g. political, religious, or sexual) and conflicts that are primarily between an individual and society are not mental disorders unless the deviance or conflict results from a dysfunction in the individual, as described above' (italics mine). This definition has nothing about a *response*; there is no requirement for a triggering event(s) or cause(s). Instead, we read of the clinical features being related to a hand-waving generalization: 'dysfunction in the psychological, biological or developmental processes underlying mental functioning'. There is no explicit requirement for any kind of objective agent triggering the mental disorder.

7. I should clarify the distinction between behavioural risk factors for a disease and making behaviour itself a disorder. Someone who drinks excessive alcohol over a long period could qualify

for the DSM 'alcohol use disorder' (as well as 'alcohol intoxication' when they get drunk). These disorders are simply their chosen behaviours; there is no distinction between the behaviour and the disorder. However, such individuals also put themselves at risk of the physical illness consequences of such heavy drinking, such as liver cirrhosis. The cirrhotic disease is not equivalent to the drinking behaviour; rather the drinking is a major risk factor for cirrhosis. It is possible to get cirrhosis without such drinking behaviour, and developing cirrhosis is not inevitable even in very heavy drinkers. Smoking is a similarly strong risk factor for lung cancer, and clearly smoking is not identified with the disease and consequent illness (although tobacco use disorder is in DSM). There are other behavioural risk factors, such as overeating and lack of exercise. These are related to a range of diseases, such as diabetes and coronary heart disease. However, the key point is that the cirrhotic disease or lung cancer or heart disease that made someone ill is not the same as the risk factor behaviour. The risky behaviour merely increases the likelihood of getting the disease. The problem with the DSM mental disorder definition is that it identifies behaviours as disorders.

8. I use 'bad' here broadly. A behaviour ('disorder') in DSM may be morally bad (sinful), e.g. pyromania and paedophilic disorder; or bad meaning unpleasant, but not sinful, e.g. hair pulling disorder; or bad meaning harmful, e.g. tobacco use disorder.

9. I am not here equating all the behaviour disorders in DSM with sin, but some of them are a medicalization of sinful behaviour.

10. Owen Whooley, 'Nosological Reflections: The Failure of DSM-5, the Emergence of RDoC, and the Decontextualization of Mental Distress', *Society and Mental Health* (2014), vol. 4(2): 92–110; doi:10.1177/2156869313519114, p. 93.

11. S. A. Martin, M. Boucher, J. M. Wright and V. Saini, 'Mild Hypertension in People at Low Risk', *BMJ* (2014); doi:10.1136/bmj.g5432.

12. The *DSM-IV* definition criterion F stated, 'No definition adequately specifies precise boundaries for the concept of "mental disorder"'; *DSM-5* has a lengthy section making this same point. But the problem is that by removing objective causation DSM discourages thinking about the context, for example about the plausible impact of stresses on all of us and what is a normal reaction.

13. D. J. Stein, K. A. Philips, D. Bolton, K. W. M. Fulford, J. Z. Sadler, K. S. Kendler, 'What Is a Mental/Psychiatric Disorder? From DSM-IV to DSM-V', *Psychological Medicine* (2010), 40(11): 1759–1765.

14. A case presentation is where a patient's personal history of mental illness and current problems are presented formally to an audience. If, as here, the audience includes staff who are not part of psychiatric services (doctors, nurses and so on), the details are carefully made anonymous so that the case (a rather impersonal term, I grant) cannot be identified.

4. Freud and the unconscious

1. Terms used for this 'below (or under) conscious awareness' are 'subconscious' or 'unconscious'. The former refers to mental activity just below conscious awareness, which may pop in and out of such awareness, while the latter indicates activity that rarely, if ever, rises to the conscious level.

2. Henri F. Ellenberger, *The Discovery of the Unconscious: The History and Evolution of Dynamic Psychiatry* (Basic Books, 1970).

3. Broadly speaking, there are two approaches to psychotherapy. One postulates that psychological problems and mental illnesses are due to forces emerging from the unconscious

mind. Freud is the most famous proponent. But there are many other schools with different models and approaches to therapy, such as from Adler, Jung and Klein. The idea they share is that dynamic forces from the unconscious shape all our behaviour. I will use the term 'Freudian' for them all. The second broad type of psychotherapy, such as 'cognitive-behavioural therapy', focuses externally on current patterns of thinking, behaviour and relationships, and does not seek to delve into the unconscious mind.

4. Ellenberger, *Discovery of the Unconscious*.

5. J. Hoenig, 'Schizophrenia', in German Berrios and Roy Porter (eds.), *A History of Clinical Psychiatry: The Origin and History of Psychiatric Disorders* (Athlone Press, 1995), p. 344.

6. Andrew Scull, *Hysteria: The Disturbing History* (Oxford University Press, 2009), pp. 176–177.

7. See ch. 7, 'Sigmund Freud and Psychoanalysis', in Ellenberger, *Discovery of the Unconscious*, p. 448.

8. Ibid., p. 549.

9. Karl Popper, *Conjectures and Refutations: The Growth of Scientific Knowledge* (Routledge, 2002), p. 49.

10. Ibid., p. 50.

11. See Gerald L. Klerman, 'The Psychiatric Patient's Right to Effective Treatment: Implications of *Osheroff v. Chestnut Lodge*', *American Journal of Psychiatry* (Apr 1990) 147(4): 409–418. See also Edward Shorter, *A History of Psychiatry: From the Era of the Asylum to the Age of Prozac* (John Wiley and Sons, 1997), pp. 309–310.

12. See for example Shorter, *A History of Psychiatry*, and Andrew Scull, *Madness: A Very Short Introduction* (Oxford University Press, 2011).

13. R. T. France, *The Gospel of Matthew*, New International Commentary on the New Testament (Eerdmans, 2007), pp. 703–705.

5. Stress and culture

1. Ben Shephard, *A War of Nerves: Soldiers and Psychiatrists, 1914–1994* (Random House, 2002), pp. 144, 165.
2. Ibid., p. 2.
3. Ibid., p. 49.
4. It is difficult even to phrase a question such as this because it seems to imply conscious planning. This illustrates the difficulty of discussing this complex topic.
5. Harold Merskey, *The Analysis of Hysteria: Understanding Conversion and Dissociation* (Royal College of Psychiatrists, 1995), p. 47.
6. Edward Shorter, *From Paralysis to Fatigue: A History of Psychsomatic Illness in the Modern Era* (The Free Press, 1992).
7. Ibid., pp. ix–x.
8. Those with a knowledge of Greek will recognize that the word 'hysteria' is derived from the Greek for womb or uterus (*hysteron*), indicating its strong association with the female sex. This association was largely self-fulfilling since men with similar symptoms were given different diagnostic labels, such as neurasthenia (exhausted nerves). Not having wombs, men couldn't have hysteria, or so it was widely believed (before shell shock).
9. As with others writing in this area, it is not possible to avoid using hysteria without references to earlier works becoming cumbersome due to repeated qualification. Instead of these, I have opted where possible to use the term 'psychosomatic' because it fits well with the biblical view of humankind, as outlined in this book, especially in chapter 1, and because it is used and recognized within medicine.
10. Andrew Scull, *Hysteria: The Disturbing History* (Oxford University Press, 2009), p. 93.
11. Simon Wessely, 'Neurasthenia and Fatigue Syndromes', in German Berrios and Roy Porter (eds.), *A History of Clinical*

Psychiatry: The Origin and History of Psychiatric Disorders (Athlone Press, 1995), p. 523.

12. Ian Hacking, *Mad Travelers: Reflections on the Reality of Transient Mental Illnesses* (Harvard University Press, 1998).

13. Almost always these travellers were men. As we noted above (n. 8), men were not usually allowed the diagnosis of hysteria and so had 'fugues'.

14. Hacking, *Mad Travelers*, p. 49.

15. Ibid., p. 50.

6. Personal responsibility and mental illness

1. Louis Berkhof, *Systematic Theology* (Banner of Truth, 1958), p. 231.

2. Andrew Sims, 'What Is Mental Disorder?', in Dominic Beer and Nigel Pocock (eds.), *Mad, Bad or Sad? A Christian Approach to Antisocial Behaviour and Mental Disorder* (Christian Medical Fellowship, 2006), p. 8.

3. Wayne Grudem, *Systematic Theology: An Introduction to Biblical Doctrine* (Inter-Varsity Press, 1994), p. 490.

4. See Christopher J. H. Wright, *The Message of Ezekiel: A New Heart and a New Spirit*, The Bible Speaks Today (Inter-Varsity Press, 2001). See pp. 181–196 for a helpful overview of this passage.

5. It is sometimes claimed that this teaching in Ezekiel 18 is inconsistent with the second commandment in Exodus 20:4–6 and Deuteronomy 5:8–10, where we read that the Lord says he punishes the children for the sins of the fathers to the third and fourth generations. Such an interpretation of the second commandment, which understood this to mean that innocent children were to be punished for the sins of their fathers and grandfathers, would also make Moses contradict himself, since in Deuteronomy 24:16 he wrote, 'Parents are not to be put to death for their children, nor children put to death for

their parents; each will die for their own sin.' Rather, Ezekiel's message is in line with this warning and with a proper interpretation of the second commandment. Douglas Stuart comments, 'This explanatory section of the second commandment, with its assertion that God is "jealous . . . punishing the children for the sins of the fathers" has been widely misunderstood . . . this oft repeated theme speaks of God's determination to punish successive generations for committing the same sins they learned from their parents. In other words, God will not say, "I won't punish this generation for what they are doing to break my covenant because, after all, they merely learned it from their parents who did it too."' See Douglas K. Stuart, *The New American Commentary on Exodus* (Broadman & Holman, 2006), p. 454. The second commandment is entirely consistent with Ezekiel's point and complements the wider conclusions that people should not be exonerated from sin because of bad parenting or bad genes.

6. Tremper Longman III, *The Book of Ecclesiastes*, New International Commentary on the Old Testament (Eerdmans, 1998), p. 219.

7. Norman L. Geisler, *If God, Why Evil? A New Way to Think about the Question* (Bethany House Publishers, 2011), ch. 8, Kindle edition.

8. Although it is possible that the meaning is merely that the child is old enough to distinguish good and bad tastes, commentators generally agree that the moral interpretation is the correct one. See, for example, J. Alec Motyer, *The Prophecy of Isaiah* (Inter-Varsity Press, 1993), p. 86, and Edward J. Young, *The Book of Isaiah* (Eerdmans, 1992), pp. 291–292.

9. Douglas K. Stuart, *Hosea–Jonah* (Word Books, 1987), pp. 506–508.

10. To be clear, we are looking here at individual guilt before God for specific acts. Everyone is held guilty before God for Adam's sin and so needs redemption by Jesus Christ.
11. The McNaughton rules are rarely used nowadays and are strictly applied only to murder cases.

7. Drugs, ECT and psychotherapy

1. Technically these are 'randomized, double-blind, parallel-group, placebo-controlled trials'. Details are beyond the scope of this book. For those interested, there are several highly readable books on this. John Diamond, *Snake Oil and Other Preoccupations* (Vintage, 2001) and Simon Singh and Edzard Ernst, *Trick or Treatment? Alternative Medicine on Trial* (Corgi, 2009) both focus on medical research that exposes the claims of alternative medicine. Ben Goldacre, *Bad Pharma: How Medicine Is Broken, and How We Can Fix It* (Fourth Estate, 2013) and David Healy, *Pharmageddon* (University of California Press, 2013) justly criticize the behaviour of large drug companies who over-claim the benefits of drugs and sometimes hide their harms.
2. Blinding is a problem for many treatments, such as psychotherapies, because you can't provide the treatment without people knowing who is receiving the therapy. The best studies use clever approaches to reduce the bias that arises when there is no blinding.
3. S. P. Roose, B. R. Rutherford, M. M. Wall, M. E. Thase, 'Practising Evidence-Based Medicine in an Era of High Placebo Response: Number Needed to Treat Reconsidered', *British Journal of Psychiatry* (2016) 208(5): 416–420.
4. B. R. Rutherford, J. Tandler, P. J. Brown, J. R. Sneed, S. P. Roose, 'Clinic Visits in Late-Life Depression Trials: Effects on Signal Detection and Therapeutic Outcome', *The American Journal of Geriatric Psychiatry: Official Journal of the American Association for Geriatric Psychiatry* (2014) 22(12): 1452–1461.

5. ADHD (also known as ADD, attention-deficit disorder) involves persistent inattention and overactivity in children, which interferes with their development. Like depression, it is a real illness but one that is overdiagnosed and thus whose numbers have been hugely inflated.

6. The Hebrew and Greek words for 'beer' are translated in different ways.

7. J. P. Louw and Eugene Albert Nida (eds.), *Greek-English Lexicon of the New Testament: Based on Semantic Domains* (United Bible Societies, 1989), p. 77.

8. Ibid.

9. Joel B. Green, *The Gospel of Luke*, New International Commentary on the New Testament (Eerdmans, 1997), p. 75.

10. John Calvin, *Commentary on the Book of Psalms* (Baker, 1989), p. 155.

11. ECT Review Group, 'Efficacy and Safety of Electroconvulsive Therapy in Depressive Disorders: A Systematic Review and Meta-Analysis', *The Lancet* (2003) 361(9360): 799–808.

12. Max Fink, 'Electroconvulsive Therapy', in Michael Gelder, Nancy Andreasen, Juan Lopez-Ibor Jr and John Geddes (eds.), *New Oxford Textbook of Psychiatry* (Oxford University Press, 2012), pp. 1251–1260.

13. Ibid.

14. Cited in Edward Shorter, *A History of Psychiatry: From the Era of the Asylum to the Age of Prozac* (John Wiley and Sons, 1997), p. 312.

15. J. C. Jakobsen, J. L. Hansen, O. J. Storebø, E. Simonsen and C. Gluud, 'The Effects of Cognitive Therapy Versus "No Intervention" for Major Depressive Disorder', *PLoS ONE* (electronic resource) (2011); 6(12): e28299.

16. J. C. Jakobsen, J. L. Hansen, E. Simonsen and C. Gluud, 'The Effect of Interpersonal Psychotherapy and Other

Psychodynamic Therapies Versus "Treatment as Usual" in Patients with Major Depressive Disorder', *PloS ONE* 2011; 6(4): e19044.

17. Will van der Hart and Rob Waller, *The Worry Book: Finding a Path to Freedom* (Inter-Varsity Press, 2011); Chris Williams, Paul Richards and Ingrid Whitton, *I'm Not Supposed to Feel Like This: A Christian Self-Help Approach to Depression and Anxiety* (Hodder & Stoughton, 2002).

18. R. A. Gotink, P. Chu, J. J. Busschbach, H. Benson, G. L. Fricchione and M. G. Hunink, 'Standardised Mindfulness-Based Interventions in Healthcare: An Overview of Systematic Reviews and Meta-Analyses of RCTs', *PloS ONE* (2015) 10(4): e0124344.

19. Ibid.

20. For example, in two high-quality reviews: 117 antidepressant trials versus 8 CBT trials, involving 25,928 subjects versus 719 subjects. A. Cipriani, T. A. Furukawa, G. Salanti et al., 'Comparative Efficacy and Acceptability of 12 New-Generation Antidepressants: A Multiple-Treatments Meta-Analysis', *The Lancet* (2009) 373(9665): 746–758; J. C. Jakobsen, J. L. Hansen, O. J. Storebø, E. Simonsen, C. Gluud, 'The Effects of Cognitive Therapy Versus "No Intervention" for Major Depressive Disorder', *PLoS ONE* (2011) 6(12): e28299. There are many other lower-quality studies of the effects of both CBT and medication on depression. The same argument applies to medication and CBT for other mental illnesses. Both are effective, but there is more good-quality evidence supporting medication.

21. J. Scott and A. H. Young, 'Psychotherapies Should Be Assessed for Both Benefit and Harm', *British Journal of Psychiatry* (2016) 208(3): 208–209.

22. N. Gartrell, J. Herman, S. Olarte, M. Feldstein and R. Localio, 'Psychiatrist-Patient Sexual Contact: Results of a National

Survey. I: Prevalence', *American Journal of Psychiatry* (1986) 143(9): 1126–1131.

23. D. J. Nutt and M. Sharpe, 'Uncritical Positive Regard? Issues in the Efficacy and Safety of Psychotherapy', *Journal of Psychopharmacology* (2008) 22(1): 3–6.

8. Psychosomatic illnesses

1. Andrew Scull, *Hysteria: The Disturbing History* (Oxford University Press, 2009), p. 102.

2. 'Neurosis' and 'neurotic' are highly loaded words. The same is true of 'hysteria' and 'hysterical'. I have chosen to avoid using the former, wherever possible, because it is difficult to do so without stigmatizing the people to whom such labels may be applied. As earlier, I restrict 'hysteria' to historical works using that term.

3. Simon Wessely, 'Neurasthenia and Fatigue Syndromes' (clinical section), in G. Berrios and R. Porter (eds.), *A History of Clinical Psychiatry: The Origin and History of Psychiatric Disorders* (Athlone Press, 1995), p. 524.

4. Ian Hacking, *Mad Travelers: Reflections on the Reality of Transient Mental Illnesses* (Harvard University Press, 1998), p. 8.

5. Studies I am familiar with show this. In the IMPACT study in the USA counsellors in primary care used these steps to improve the care of people with milder forms of depressive illness: J. Unutzer et al., 'Collaborative Care Management of Late-Life Depression in the Primary Care Setting: A Randomized Controlled Trial', *Jama* (2002) 288(22): 2836–2845. In India in the MANAS study, lay health counsellors again used similar steps to benefit people with psychosomatic illnesses: V. Patel et al., 'Effectiveness of an Intervention Led by Lay Health Counsellors for Depressive and Anxiety Disorders in Primary Care in Goa, India (MANAS): A Cluster Randomised Controlled Trial', *The Lancet* (2010); 376(9758):

2086–2095. Although these therapists had some minimal training and supervision, church leaders benefit from having more relevant experience and knowledge than the therapists in these trials.

6. The first three steps here are the core elements of what is referred to as 'behavioural activation'. Engaging individuals in supportive relationships, encouraging them to work and to take regular exercise are recognized as activating people so that their psychosomatic symptoms improve.

7. Recent studies report a reduction in the numbers of people with dementia, and earlier studies looking at schizophrenia reported improvements before antipsychotic drugs were available, due in part to improvements in diet and living conditions. With other mental illnesses, especially psychosomatic ones, such evidence is difficult to provide because of the large changes in definitions we discussed earlier. You need consistent diagnosis over time to see such effects.

8. In England IAPT services were introduced about a decade ago to make psychotherapies more widely available. IAPT is a clumsy acronym, which stands for Improving Access to Psychological Treatments.

9. Will van der Hart and Rob Waller, *The Worry Book: Finding a Path to Freedom* (Inter-Varsity Press, 2011); Chris Williams, Paul Richards and Ingrid Whitton, *I'm Not Supposed to Feel Like This: A Christian Approach to Depression and Anxiety* (Hodder & Stoughton, 2002).

10. Anorexia nervosa is the medical term for what is commonly just called 'anorexia'. Anorexia simply means 'not eating' and is of course common in many illnesses. Use of 'nervosa' clarifies that the cause of the anorexia is psychological.

11. BMI (body mass index) is the standard measure for assessing healthy bodyweight. It is calculated by dividing weight (in

kilogrammes) by height (in metres) squared. The healthy range for bodyweight is 18–25 kg/m^2.

12. Fibromyalgia is here an example of a psychosomatic illness that is usually not dealt with by psychiatrists and not regarded as a mental illness. People have fluctuating aches and pains in their muscles and fatigue, but associated prominent mental symptoms too. Sadly, the importance of the psychological contribution and emotional symptoms is often missed.

9. Severe mental illnesses: schizophrenia, dementia, bipolar disorder and depression

1. SMI is usually used in the singular (severe mental illness). I use the plural, as the focus here is on the several illnesses in this category.

2. Andrew Sims, in *New Oxford Textbook of Psychiatry* (Oxford University Press, 2012), section 1.7, p. 50.

3. Dawkins has followed the sad history of many others who have taken technical psychiatric labels and used them as terms of abuse to hurl at people they disagree with. Thus, 'mad', 'insane', 'moron', 'idiot' and others began in psychiatry before becoming insults used in invective.

4. Stefan Leucht et al., 'Comparative Efficacy and Tolerability of 15 Antipsychotic Drugs in Schizophrenia: A Multiple-Treatments Meta-Analysis', *The Lancet* (2013) 382(9896): 951–962; doi:0.1016/S0140-6736(13)60733-3.

5. Ibid.

6. Here and elsewhere I simply state the most common or important side effects (adverse effects) of the drugs. These are the sorts of potential problems I discuss with patients. The full list of side effects for any drug is listed on the insert that comes with the medication prescription.

7. S. Jauhar et al., 'Cognitive-Behavioural Therapy for the Symptoms of Schizophrenia: Systematic Review and

Meta-Analysis with Examination of Potential Bias', *British Journal of Psychiatry* (2014) 204(1): 20–29; doi:10.1192/bjp.bp.112.116285.

8. These are usually called behavioural and psychological symptoms of dementia (BPSD) by health professionals.

9. Strictly speaking, manic depression (originally manic-depressive insanity or MDI)) was a different concept from today's bipolar disorder. It included depressive and bipolar disorders. Later it was narrowed and came to be used interchangeably with bipolar disorder.

10. Again, I am using the robust figures for narrowly defined bipolar disorder. As with all other mental illnesses, larger figures are reported when the criteria for diagnosis are broadened. See Peter R. Joyce, 'Epidemiology of Mood Disorders', in Michael Gelder, Nancy Andreasen, Juan Lopez-Ibor Jr and John Geddes (eds.), in *New Oxford Textbook of Psychiatry* (Oxford University Press, 2012), section 4.5.4, p. 646.

11. John R. Geddes and David J. Miklowitz, 'Treatment of Bipolar Disorder', *The Lancet* (2013) 381: 1672–1682.

12. Michael E. Thase et al., 'The Promise of Cognitive Behavior Therapy for Treatment of Severe Mental Disorders: A Review of Recent Developments', *World Psychiatry* (2014) 13(3): 244–250; doi:10.1002/wps.20149.

13. From Lewis Carroll, *Through the Looking-Glass*, ch. 6, 'Humpty Dumpty'.

14. M. G. Hamer and D. Batty, 'Antidepressant Medication Use and Future Risk of Cardiovascular Disease: The Scottish Health Survey', *European Heart Journal* (2011) 32(4): 437–442. See also M. Olfson and S. C. Marcus, 'National Patterns in Antidepressant Medication Treatment', *Archives of General Psychiatry* (2009) 66(8): 848–856.

15. Edward Shorter, *How Everyone Became Depressed: The Rise and Fall of the Nervous Breakdown* (Oxford University Press, 2013).

16. In the late 1970s the leading figures preparing for *DSM-III* originally included a minor depression category. However, insurance companies in the USA would not pay for treatment for any condition deemed 'minor'. So the term was not included in *DSM-III* in 1980 and hasn't been in successive editions. Instead, 'major depression' has been made to cover both major and minor forms of depression. This history is recounted in Edward Shorter's *How Everyone Became Depressed*, *passim*.

17. CBT for depression has been extensively studied and there are some helpful guides written from a Christian perspective: Will van der Hart and Rob Waller, *The Worry Book: Finding a Path to Freedom* (Inter-Varsity Press, 2011); Chris Williams, Paul Richards and Ingrid Whitton, *I'm Not Supposed to Feel Like This: A Christian Approach to Depression and Anxiety* (Hodder & Stoughton, 2002).

18. N. A. Khin, Y-F Chen, Y. Yang, P. Yang and T. P. Laughren, 'Exploratory Analyses of Efficacy Data from Major Depressive Disorder Trials Submitted to the US Food and Drug Administration in Support of New Drug Applications', *Journal of Clinical Psychiatry* (2011) 72(4): 464–472.

19. This lack of movement is called psychomotor retardation and again reflects our psychosomatic wholeness.